**David Barmore Productions**
P.O. Box 250, Todd Road
Stamford, NY 12167

In Fitness and In Health:
The No-Nonsense Guide to Diet, Exercise and Disease Prevention
Fourth Revised Edition

Managing Editor: Hal Walter
Copy Editor: Mary Lyn Koval
Cover Designer: Kathy Fulton
Text Designer: Diane French
Proofreader: Teresa Cutler
Illustrators: Diane French, Monica Sheehan

Printed in the United States
Library of Congress Control Number: 2002106919
ISBN: 0-9679450-1-1

# The
# NO-NONSENSE
## Guide
### to
## Diet,
## Exercise
### and
## Disease Prevention

**Dr. Philip Maffetone**

*"Now I see the secret*

*of the making*

*of the best persons.*

*It is to grow in the open air,*

*and to eat and sleep*

*with the earth."*

— Walt Whitman, *Leaves of Grass*

# Table of Contents

# Introduction

We are entering a new era in health care, as the responsibility for personal health shifts from the health-care system back to each of us. It's a time when we demand higher quality of life now and for the future. In this age of true prevention, we seek to avoid or postpone cancer, heart disease and Alzheimer's rather than settle for early detection. We would rather be full of life in our "golden years" than spend a decade or more at the end of life in dysfunction. The tools to do this are contained in this newly rewritten and greatly expanded fourth edition of *In Fitness and In Health* — a book first printed in 1990.

From that very first edition, I sought to share my experiences with improving health as a balance of art and science. This stemmed from my clinical practice in complementary medicine, which began in 1977, and — previous to that — being a patient. The art facet entails a unique understanding of fitness and health. I compiled the actual science through extensive research. In this book I combine this art with this science in hopes of helping you to fully understand and simplify many of the complex mechanisms of fitness and health.

I have worked with patients from all walks of life, from the most healthy to the most frail, from professional athletes to couch potatoes. Many had unique imbalances that not only caused dysfunction, but detracted from their quality of life, reducing what I call "human performance." Many of these problems were the result of dietary and nutritional imbalances, and others stemmed from deficiencies in the aerobic system or the stress-coping mechanisms. It was clear that addressing these problems immediately and individually was the key not only to improving health in the short term, but also avoiding serious disease in the long run.

This reorganized and extensively updated edition addresses steps you can take to improve your health and fitness for a better quality of life now, and a longer life and higher human performance in your later years. It opens by defining key issues, terms and philosophies important in understanding how to achieve a balance of health and fitness, and optimal human performance. Since your health is so dependent upon your diet, the second section of this book extensively discusses diet and nutrition, with some of the material challenging many long-held popular beliefs. Exercise is basic not only to fitness but also to health, and thus the third section of this book discusses developing or modifying an exercise program most appropriate for your needs. Lastly, the section on self-health management ties together all the wisdom in the book. Included is the newest information that is scientifically based and clinically relevant, presented in a user-friendly format, with specific actions you can take to understand and prevent the most dangerous diseases facing modern humankind. By correcting and diverting seemingly subtle problems, you can prevent disease, modify the aging process, and drastically improve the quality of your life.

Today genetics is a hot topic, but your lifestyle can more often offset unhealthy genetic predispositions. The truth is you have more control over this lifestyle — through diet, nutrition, stress control, exercise and other factors — than you probably ever imagined. The remedies for the greatest of ailments have been with us all along. By redirecting and rethinking your responsibility in health care, you can immediately begin reaping the benefits.

While many so-called health programs come and go, there is no one approach for everyone, except one that teaches how to individualize health and fitness to meet each of our unique needs. This book will help you do just that — determine which lifestyle factors best match your particular needs. Many may be just the opposite of conventional wisdom or what you are currently doing. By the end of the book you will know not only how to live most healthfully, but also how to die most successfully.

You'll want to read this book from beginning to end, then continuously refer to it. Each time you read from it you'll understand more about the complexity of this puzzle we call the human body. In doing so, you'll want to share the information with friends and family, perhaps influencing others in their quest for better health and fitness.

Good health and fitness forever!

—— Dr. Phil Maffetone

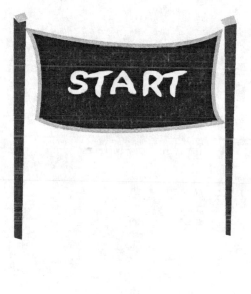

# 1 Defining Health and Fitness

It was the summer of 1976, and I wanted to watch the Olympic sprinters in Montreal. I was in a hospital bed with an undiagnosed illness that had caused me to drop 60 pounds in less than a year. Now, weighing only 97 pounds, I was barely able to reach the switch for the TV and too weak to turn it on. The nurse came in to help me. While watching the Olympic games, I remembered the days when I was a national-class sprinter. And I wondered how my health could so rapidly deteriorate.

The road to full recovery from that illness was long and required that I learn more about how my body works. In a sense I'm still on that road, continually assessing my diet, nutrition, physical activity and lifestyle in order to stay healthy.

By tuning in more closely to my body's needs after my illness I began to see the immediate benefits of improved health and also began to feel well for the first time in several years. During this period I began a walking program. In April 1980, I found myself admiring the finishers of the Boston Marathon, thinking that these runners must be really healthy in order to run more than 26 miles. As I watched the marathoners finish I developed a desire to test my own health. I had been walking regularly for more than two years. The New York City Marathon was six months away and that seemed like plenty of time to train. After all, I mused, I ran in high school and in college.

It was a cool, overcast morning as I began my journey to the New York City Marathon. The race started with a cannon blast so loud it shook the Verrazano Bridge. The crowd of 18,000 runners began to move and I was among them, ready to prove to myself that I really was healthy.

All went well through the first 10 miles. The excitement swept me along at a slightly quicker pace than planned, yet I felt great. As expected, by 15 miles I felt tired but was able to continue. Within the next couple of miles, however, I began to shiver. Despite drinking plenty of water, I felt dehydrated. And I was craving cotton candy.

At 18 miles, I stopped to check my feet. They were numb, and I wanted to be sure they were still there. "My hamstrings are cramping," I said out loud. Suddenly I realized I wasn't thinking rationally and all I could remember was my goal to finish the race and prove my health.

Alarmed by how bad I looked, two men tried to take me off the course. But I wouldn't stop. Somehow, I fought my way onward. I have very little memory of those last few miles, but I'll always remember the finale. A minor collision with a TV camera in Central Park made me realize I was close to the end of the race. As the pain became more intense the crowds got louder, and for the first time in quite a while I had a clear view — the finish line.

A medal was hung around my neck, and I cried. I thought the lesson was over, but I would soon be struck by a more meaningful one. The next moment I discovered myself in the first-aid tent. It looked like a war zone. There were casualties all around me. Doctors and nurses were running around. People on cots groaned in pain. Ambulances came and went.

Looking around I had to wonder: "Are these people really healthy?" I realized then that running the marathon had not proven my health at all. I was fit enough to run 26.2 miles. But clearly fitness was something quite different from health. The next morning, sore but happy, I pondered my new goal to improve my health. Achieving this would not be so simple as running a marathon. Optimal health would be something that I would continually strive to attain for the rest of my life.

So the real lesson from my marathon experience was not one of proving health, but rather that I became fit enough to run a marathon. Clearly this had nothing to do with my health. *Fitness* and *health*, though many think the terms are interchangeable, are actually two different, but mutually dependent states.

Later, in treating patients who were very athletic, I would see individuals who were very fit but also quite unhealthy; injuries, illness and other unhealthy conditions often accompanied their quests to be faster or go farther. Clearly, some athletes would be healthier had they stayed couch potatoes! On the other hand, I saw many sedentary people who attempted to get healthy without an adequate level of fitness — also a condition that was not ideal. The main reason for the dysfunction in both types of patients is an imbalance between fitness and health. Let us define these two important terms as follows:

**Fitness:** The ability to perform physical activity. You define the limits of your fitness; you can walk a mile a day or train for the Ironman Triathlon.

**Health:** The optimal balance of all systems of the body — the nervous, muscular, skeletal, circulatory, digestive, lymphatic, hormonal, mental, emotional and all other systems.

Improving fitness is associated with physical activity. Only a couple of generations ago, most people were naturally active, working hard physically to accomplish their daily chores. Today, we have escalators, microwaves and remote controls. Some people drive around a parking lot for 10 minutes to get a parking space closer to the door. Others wait minutes for an elevator just to go to the first floor. We can fulfill most of our needs literally at the push of a button. This radical change from a vigorous to an inactive lifestyle has taken place, genetically speaking, in a very short time frame. The human body can't adapt to such a major change without dire consequences. Our relative inactivity has resulted in an overweight society and an entire host of other functional problems such as blood-sugar problems, fatigue and low-back pain. This is followed by increased rates of diabetes, heart disease, cancer and other diseases. Dysfunction and disease are, in large part, due to not taking care of the body.

Since most of us have lost the natural tendency to be active like our very recent ancestors, we must satisfy that need artificially, by exercising. Without some fitness activity, you can't improve your level of health. And don't forget the issue of balance; too much activity can also impair your health.

Steps to improving your health may include eating real foods rather than processed, obtaining real vitamins or other nutrients from foods rather than synthetic supplements, and controlling stress. These and other specifics are discussed throughout this book.

With my realization that fitness and health are two different states also came the conclusion that these states are elements of an even larger concept — *human performance*. When health and fitness are balanced, the result is optimal human performance. We often associate human performance with the fulfillment of some athletic feat, like winning an Olympic gold medal. But in the true sense, human performance pertains to all aspects of life, including personal, family, social and work functions. Performance pertains to either physical or mental activities, or both. The benefits of improved human performance include increased energy, productivity and creativity, and better relationships with people. In my practice I had the pleasure and excitement to actually see people improve their human performance, and thus succeed at whatever their primary goal in life was at the time. These goals included winning the Ironman Triathlon, achieving career success, and being the best-possible parent. The secret to reaching any of these goals is optimal human performance, and its foundation is balanced fitness and health. Thus, we have this definition of human performance and the following equation:

**Human Performance:** The balance between health and fitness that allows a person to achieve success in all areas of life.

**Fitness + Health = Human Performance**

This is a relatively simple concept to understand, but it's important to note that this equation is not one-directional, as its effects are actually cyclical and exponential. In other words, increased human performance can, in return, also bring about even greater improvements in the foundational elements of fitness and heath. Thus, as you improve your fitness and health, thereby improving your human performance, this additional human performance can fuel even further improvements in your health and fitness. There's virtually no end to this cycle, meaning that a person can achieve virtually unlimited physical and mental energy. It's really just a matter of how far you are willing to go to improve your fitness and your health.

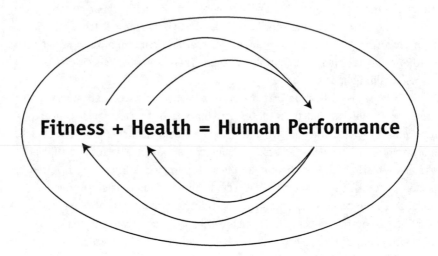

**Fitness + Health = Human Performance**

# 2 Unlimited Physical and Mental Energy

Your body must produce large amounts of energy for all physical and mental activities. With proper balance between health and fitness, your body will have no trouble meeting the energy requirements for optimal human performance.

But where does this energy come from? The answer is both simple and complex. Basically, your energy comes from the sun. Light energy from the sun comes to earth and is converted to chemical energy in plants through the process of photosynthesis. We eat the plants, and many of us eat animals that eat plants. The chemical energy we take in is converted to mechanical energy that fuels our physical and mental activities, enabling us to move, work and exercise. More directly, the energy produced by the body comes from the foods we eat. This energy is obtained from the basic macronutrients in food — carbohydrate, fat and protein. Though many foods contain all three, there's usually a predominance of one of these in each food. The following chart lists some common examples.

| Carbohydrates | Fats | Proteins |
|---|---|---|
| Bread, sugar, rice, pasta, fruit and fruit juice, cereal | Oils, butter, high-fat cheeses, egg yolk | Meat, fish, poultry, eggs, cheese (curds & whey) |

The majority of energy is produced from two of these food groups — carbohydrate and fat. Only a small amount, up to 15 percent of total energy, is produced from protein (by conversion of certain amino acids into glucose). All three food groups are converted into energy in two steps. First, they are broken down in the intestine and absorbed into the blood: as glucose from carbohydrates, fatty acids from fats, and amino acids from protein.

In the second step, the blood ultimately carries these elements to the cells, where the molecules of glucose, fatty acids and amino acids are further broken down. The hydrogen atom, the common building block of all three food groups, is released as a result of further chemical breakdown. This atom contains one electron that is highly charged with energy. This electron is finally converted to a substance called ATP, which the body uses as energy.

To get even more specific, we could say the body's energy comes from hydrogen's electron. Carbohydrates, fats and proteins each have different amounts of hydrogen molecules, and potential energy. Fats have by far the most hydrogen, one reason we can get much more energy from fats. Fats can provide more than twice the energy you get from either carbohydrates or proteins.

Where does all this energy-generating activity take place? Mostly it is produced by your metabolism in the aerobic muscle fibers, which primarily use fat as a fuel. When these muscles are functioning optimally, you can derive even more energy from fat. In fact, up to 90 percent of your energy at any given time can come from fat, and the energy supply is virtually endless — the average lean person has enough stored fat to endure a 1,000-mile trek!

The more energy you derive from fat the better your fitness, health and human performance. By improving your fat-burning system, you'll improve metabolic efficiency and have more physical and mental energy. In addition, your body will store less fat, and you'll maintain a more stable blood-sugar level because you won't need as much sugar for energy.

When you don't produce the required amount of energy from fat, your body instead relies too heavily on sugar, usually producing a symptom — fatigue. Fatigue is one of the most common complaints heard by doctors. It comes in physical and mental forms, or in a combination of both. Some people say they just can't perform as they did when they were younger. But age is no excuse for a lack of energy. Physical fatigue may strike at a particular time of the day, or it may make you feel exhausted from the time you awaken. You may feel you don't have the energy to do extra chores, go out at night or even get up in the morning. Mental fatigue is also common, making it difficult to think clearly or make decisions. This can affect anyone from students to executives.

For you to avoid fatigue and instead access unlimited energy from your fat-burning system, two things must occur. First, you need to develop and utilize the body's aerobic muscle fibers, along with the entire aerobic system. Second, you need to provide those muscle fibers with the proper mixture of fuel that they require. These items are discussed in the coming chapters.

To maintain efficient fat-burning, you also must burn some sugar. Herein lies another example of balance. Both fat and sugar are almost always being burned for energy at all times. It's a question of how much of each we use. Right now, you may be getting half of your energy from fat and half from sugar. When you improve your aerobic system and fat-burning capabilities, you may be able to obtain 70 percent of your energy from fat and 30 percent from sugar. But many people only get 10 percent of their energy from fat, forcing a full 90 percent to come from sugar. That's a very inefficient and unhealthy way to get energy. This is the typical situation in a person who is fatigued and attempts to obtain more energy from sugar because he can't get much from fat. And since the fat is not used for energy, it is stored in the body. This book explains how to reverse this situation and improve your fat-burning system.

**Measuring Fat- and Sugar-Burning**
This mix of fuels used for energy can be measured in a person easily, and is something I have done during my years in practice and during other research. So when I say you can improve your fat-burning capability, it is because I have seen and recorded these changes in actual patients. These measurements are taken using a gas analyzer, which measures the amount of oxygen a person inhales and the amount of carbon dioxide exhaled. The ratio of carbon dioxide to oxygen gives the percentage of fat and sugar that is used for energy. This is referred to as the *respiratory quotient*, or RQ.

Measuring a person's RQ on a stationary bike or treadmill shows how the amounts of fat and sugar used for fuel adjust with changes in intensity of physical exertion. Generally, with higher physical intensity the ratio adjusts to burn more sugar and less fat. That's why for many people easy walking promotes more fat-burning than does running. However, through proper conditioning anyone can promote higher amounts of fat-burning at higher levels of physical intensity. Many athletes, in fact, are able to run at a very fast pace and still burn significant amounts of fat.

Below is a list of some patients' RQ numbers at rest and their symptoms. Take away the names, and this list could be viewed as the progression of one person who improves his or her aerobic and fat-burning systems through proper dietary adjustments and conditioning.

| Name | RQ | Complaints |
|------|-----|-----------|
| JC | 88% sugar, 12% fat | extreme fatigue, insomnia, 45 lbs. overweight |
| BK | 74% sugar, 26% fat | afternoon & evening fatigue, asthma, headaches |
| JO | 62% sugar, 38% fat | 4 p.m. fatigue, seasonal allergies, 10 lbs. overweight |
| PS | 55% sugar, 45% fat | chronic, mild knee pain, indigestion |
| MK | 42% sugar, 58% fat | occasional low-back pain |
| BE | 37% sugar, 63% fat | none |

Remember, these measurements were taken at rest, not while exercising. This reflects rates of sugar- and fat-burning that these people use for all daily activities. As you can see, the patients who burn more sugar and less fat are the most unhealthy, and have the most functional problems. These functional problems, such as weight gain, fatigue, headaches and others, are some of the problems encountered on the road to disease. On the other hand, those who rely less on sugar and who burn more fat for fuel have fewer or even no functional problems. The bottom line: Less sugar-burning and more fat-burning at any level of intensity improves health, fitness and human performance.

# 3 Assessing for Function and Preventing Disease

We've now seen how balancing your health and fitness leads to greater human performance and more production of energy for all aspects of your life. But more often than not, some piece of this equation gets out of balance. The result is dysfunction, and ultimately disease. We're all too familiar with the common diseases, such as heart disease, cancer and stroke. But how do these diseases begin? The truth is most diseases don't just happen overnight. They have their beginnings as functional problems due to some imbalance of the health and fitness equation.

## Functional Illness

There are often no particular names for various early stages of disease development. There are simply signs and symptoms, although even previous to that you get no clues that a problem is arising. These signs and symptoms, as subtle as they may be, are known as functional problems, or *functional illness*. They are sometimes referred to as pre-disease, pre-clinical or, in the case of cancer, pre-malignant. Functional illness is that gray area between optimal health and disease.

Many people have some signs and symptoms of functional illness, such as fatigue, headaches, indigestion, back pain, allergies and dozens of other complaints. Not only can functional illness be the early stage of disease, it can also interfere with present quality of life. It's not normal to have these problems; it's a sign that something is wrong. The shelves of grocery stores and pharmacies are loaded with products we use to medicate ourselves to mask these minor illnesses. But masking the problem does not make it go away, and worse yet, it turns off your body's attempt to tell you there's something wrong. These types of signs and symptoms aren't really addressed by mainstream medicine, which usually deals only with disease, the after effect of functional illness.

### Case History

*John went to the company doctor for his annual physical examination. Many tests were performed — a very complete evaluation. The next week when John returned for the results, the doctor said, "Good news, everything looks great, there's nothing wrong." True, everything from blood pressure to cholesterol, clear lungs to strong heart was great news, but John was now more confused. He asked, "Then why*

19

*do I have these headaches, and why is my energy so low? And why*
*does my stomach always hurt after eating?" The doctor had no*
*answer other than to say that he had ruled out disease.*

In ruling out disease, John's doctor performed a vital service. But it was only the first step in evaluating John's health and fitness. Though John didn't have any disease, he had symptoms that made him uncomfortable and were interfering with his quality of life. What's more, these symptoms could be pointing to bigger problems down the road. This is a common example of functional illness.

Such functional illness — or dysfunction — is often the precursor to disease. By assessing your level of function you can find and correct many problems before they become diseases. When I was in practice, a significant part of my initial examination of a patient was listening to his or her problems. I heard the main complaints of "I'm tired all day" or "my back hurts," but I more closely tuned in to other details such as waking in the middle of the night and being unable to get back to sleep, or exactly at what time of day the back felt worse, and when it was OK. Most of what I needed to know came from the patient telling me things he or she was not fully aware of. These kinds of clues, the subtle and the obvious ones, and what they mean, are called functional problems and are discussed throughout this book.

One way to know if you have a functional illness is through self-assessment. When we start listening to ourselves we will begin to get many clues. Once we have collected these clues, sorting them out becomes another art form. The most important distinction to make is in the difference between primary and secondary problems. I call this the domino effect.

The body tends to accumulate problems, often beginning with one small, seemingly minor imbalance. This problem causes another subtle imbalance, which triggers another, then several more. In the end, you get a symptom. It's like lining up a series of dominoes. All you need to do is knock down the first one and many others will fall too. What caused the last one to fall? Obviously it wasn't the one before it, or the one before that, but the first one.

The body works the same way. The initial problem is often unnoticed. It's not until some of the later "dominoes" fall that more obvious clues and symptoms appear. In the end, you get a headache, fatigue or depression — or even disease. When you try to treat the last domino — treat just the end-result symptom — the cause of the problem isn't addressed.

The first domino is the cause, or primary problem, and is often asymptomatic, meaning that you don't notice it. The next dominoes are the main complaint, or secondary problem, which produces the symptom but is merely the result of the first domino. The final domino is disease itself. Being able to differentiate between primary and secondary problems is important for all of us, including health-care professionals. The classic example of this is treating a diseased organ. A heart-bypass operation or organ replacement satisfies the end result. But what about the cause of the problem? If it's not found, how long will it take before another major problem arises, if it hasn't already?

As you become more intuitive about your health, you will begin to understand the signs and symptoms your body is providing in its desire to get your attention and your help. Once you develop your instincts, you'll be able to take responsibility to care for your own health. For those who can't or won't assess for functional illness and take appropriate actions to correct problems, there's always disease.

## Disease

*Disease* can be defined quite simply as a gross imbalance of normal body function. Disease is the end result of dysfunction expressed by signs and symptoms of something in the body that has gone wrong. Heart disease, for example, begins many years or decades before the first sign of its presence appears (the most common one, unfortunately, being death). For almost all diseases there's a build-up of imbalances, and this eventually causes the end-result disease state.

Perhaps the most important question you should ask yourself is: Are there indications of these diseases earlier, in the pre-disease state? The answer is most definitely, yes! Your body always tells you when something is going out of balance. In the case of heart disease, for example, abnormal blood cholesterol ratios or chronic inflammation, as discussed in later chapters, could be indications you are at risk. Both can be assessed through simple blood tests. These signs of dysfunction may exist years before the disease. What about even before your cholesterol goes askew? It's well known that men who develop even moderate amounts of abdominal fat are at much higher risk for a heart attack. And, symptoms like sleepiness and intestinal bloating after meals begin long before the fat begins showing up on the abdomen. Even early clues such as being overfat in childhood may be predictive.

Assessing for these signs in order to prevent disease is an important aspect of maintaining your fitness, health and human performance. In later chapters we'll discuss more specifics about assessing for functional problems and avoiding disease throughout life's journey, which I call the human race.

# 4 Welcome to the Human Race

Most people don't think of themselves as athletes or competitors. The fact is, we're all in a race: the human race. We run to work, rush through business, race through lunch, dash to the store and tear through our errands. As we get older, life seems to get more complicated rather than easier, and more time-consuming. We wonder how we'll keep up this pace for the rest of our lives. The truth is, most people don't. In the United States, the average person spends the last 12 years of life in a state of gross dysfunction, relying on others for care and just waiting to die. Many spend a lifetime of savings to maintain a few more moments of a poor-quality life. Instead of sprinting to life's finish line, most people reach it only after an agonizing death march.

Welcome to the human race. It's analogous to a very long journey, say, of 1,000 miles. If you were going to go that distance, you'd have to prepare for it, following certain rules. You'd have to find the optimal diet and nutritional program that matches your individual needs. You'd need to prepare physically. You would need to assess for dysfunction to prevent injury and disease. You would have to make lifestyle adjustments that increase your fitness, health and human performance. If your life is like a 1,000-mile journey, just how are you preparing for it?

I've actually trained an athlete who completed such an event, a 1,000-mile ultramarathon. Stu Mittleman broke the world record by more than 16 hours when he ran the New York 1,000-mile event in 1986. After 11 days and 19 hours of racing, Stu looked stronger than many people do on Friday afternoon after a week at the office. This ultramarathoner considers himself a typical and average

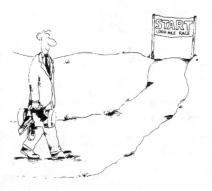

person. His training wasn't excessive. In fact, Stu called the training "excessive moderation." In many ways, the basic program Stu followed was similar to the one you can use in your life's journey.

The 1,000-mile race Stu Mittleman won was a true test of endurance. So is life. We are all endurance animals, and we must use the natural endurance we all possess by unlocking our aerobic and fat-burning systems through proper nutrition and conditioning. Most patients I've seen — athletes and non-athletes alike — have gross deficiencies in their endurance systems. They can't keep up in life's journey.

The endurance system is also called the *aerobic system*, encompassing, in part, the heart, lungs, blood vessels and aerobic muscle fibers. It's fueled by nutrients obtained from the right kinds of foods, including fats, and the right exercise. If you "turn on" this aerobic system with easy exercise and proper diet, you will burn more fat and perform well in the human race.

There's another system at work in the body, which burns mostly sugar: This is the *anaerobic system*, or short-term, speed system. This is what you use when sprinting for the train, or chasing after a toddler. It's also the system that revs up when you're under stress. Too much anaerobic activity will cause the body to burn more sugar while storing fat. This fat may accumulate in the blood vessels, abdomen or hips. Overuse of the anaerobic system will produce symptoms that may include mental and physical fatigue, moodiness, low blood sugar and recurrent or chronic injury, to name a few. If you try to get through life's journey using this system, you're apt to have a very hard time.

Aerobic- and anaerobic-system imbalances result from lifestyle habits, social trends and misinformation. Fortunately, these imbalances can be corrected. Stu Mittleman ran his 1,000-mile race by following a pre-race plan, specific to his needs. He compiled his 84-mile-per-day average with consistency, running some miles and walking others. He didn't try to do it all the first day, or even the first week. Because Stu had a plan and good preparation, nothing went wrong. That's not to say it was easy. It was hard work, but he was geared for success.

You must do the same in life's journey. It's important to avoid the dangerous tendency to "get fit" quickly or lose the excess weight in a week. Stu ran his own race, and all of us must do the same. Beyond the basic rules, everyone has individual requirements. Each of you can discover your own needs for a personal best in life's journey. While Stu ran his own race, most of the other runners ran in a random, trial-and-error style. A few days into the race, many were experiencing pain from blisters, swollen joints and extreme fatigue.

If you try to run life's race in that same random way, your race won't go well. It can be difficult relying on your natural instincts for living because they have been lost in the modern way of life. They can be retrieved through education and healthy habits. If you're prepared for life's long journey, you can achieve the same results Stu did — a world-class performance. This is a book about preparing for life's long journey. In the following sections we will discuss specifics of diet and nutrition, exercise and self-health management that can make a huge difference in your success in the human race.

I hope to see you at the finish line.

# YOU ARE WHAT YOU EAT

# 5 The Basic Recipe: Choose Your Food Wisely

In order to enjoy optimal human performance and generate unlimited amounts of energy, you must make wise decisions about the foods you eat. It's true that you are what you eat — the quality of each morsel you consume can dramatically influence the quality of your body and the quality of its performance. But as many times as you've heard that you should "eat well," you've probably also heard just as many different recommendations about what, and how much of what, to eat. Everyone has an opinion, from the popular and unhealthy low-fat approach to the faddish and unbalanced high-protein diets. Which eating plan is the right recipe for you?

Just as each of us has a different set of fingerprints, our specific requirements for carbohydrates, fats and proteins, along with the right amounts of vitamins, minerals and fiber, can vary, sometimes dramatically, from person to person. To build and maintain your health you must supply your body with the right mix of fuels and nutrients that matches your individual needs. Rigid diets that specify what foods you should and shouldn't eat don't work for a population of individuals. Some people thrive on a vegetarian diet; others need meat to be healthy. Some people have allergies to different kinds of foods, and all of us have unique food preferences. That's why one diet plan can't work for the whole population. Your job is to find out what works for you, something you'll learn in this book.

At one time, people instinctively knew what to eat. Today, we have lost that ability and instead we look to others for advice. Often this advice is misguided. In addition, large corporations spend billions of dollars telling us what we're hungry for. And it works — how many times have you seen a commercial on TV and suddenly had an intense craving for whatever was being advertised? We can't choose our meals and snacks on the advice of people who don't know our individual needs, or by what looks good in a TV commercial — that is, not if we want optimal human performance.

## The Pyramid Scheme

Remember that old joke: "Hi, I'm from the government, and I'm here to help you?" In 1992 the United States Department of Agriculture (USDA) decided its dietary guideline program known as the "four food groups" (there were really five food groups) needed improvement, and created the food pyramid. This approach advocates eating the bulk of calories from carbohydrate foods such as bread, cereal, rice and pasta, which form the base of the pyramid. From there the pyramid suggests you eat lesser amounts of vegetables and fruits, dairy products, meats and eggs. Lastly, small amounts of fats and sweets make up the tip of the pyramid.

As with much that comes out of our nation's capitol, there are a number of problems associated with this "pyramid scheme." Rather than building the pyramid using sound general recommendations of scientists and clinicians, the USDA allowed special-interest groups and lobbyists from the food industry to have their input. Thus the food pyramid turned out to be a misguided public-information program. Following this high-carbohydrate program is equivalent to eating two cups of sugar a day. Ironically, this food pyramid stands today as a figurative monument over an increasingly overweight and disease-ridden society.

Edward Siguel, M.D., Ph.D., of Boston University Medical Center, writing in the September 1995 issue of the *American Journal of Clinical Nutrition,* said justification of the USDA food pyramid is based on obsolete recommendations and is scientifically incorrect. Specific problems with the current USDA pyramid include high-glycemic carbohydrate excess, imbalances of essential fatty acids and low levels of other nutrients.

The food pyramid suggests that most foods consumed should be bread, cereal, rice and pasta — up to 11 servings a day! Most people consume carbohydrates in their processed form as white bread including rolls, bagels and crackers, processed cereals, white rice and white-flour pasta. These high-glycemic products are among the most harmful foods; they rapidly raise blood sugar and insulin and can contribute to heart disease, cancer, hypertension, diabetes and other diseases.

Additionally, certain dietary fats are essential for good health. These include omega-6 and omega-3 fats found in certain oils as discussed in following chapters. However, the current food pyramid recommends that fats be used sparingly. The importance of essential-fatty-acid (EFA) balance is not even mentioned in the USDA guidelines. According to Siguel, a slim woman eating 1,500 kilocalories (kcal) per day who faithfully follows the USDA food pyramid easily obtains 700 calories from breads, pasta and cereals. The remaining 800 calories may come from vegetables, fruits, chicken and low-fat dairy products. From these foods she cannot possibly get the 15 to 20 grams of omega-6 and omega-3 essential fatty acids required daily.

In the United States, EFA imbalance affects more than 50 million people. Following the food pyramid guidelines may have already worsened this trend. Yet the pyramid suggests eating fats sparingly. Even worse is the food pyramid recommendation promoting the use of margarine, which is often made of hydrogenated and partially hydrogenated fat; its consumption can disrupt the balance of fats and promote ill health and disease.

In addition, assessments of the food pyramid diet made by NutrAnalysis, Inc., show low and borderline levels of many vitamins and minerals. A sample diet of a 52-year-old woman who consumed 1,600 calories based on the food pyramid had levels below the recommended daily allowances (RDA) of pantothenic acid, vitamins B6, B12 and E, biotin and the minerals chromium, copper, iodine, iron, magnesium, manganese, sodium and zinc. Borderline RDA levels included those in folic acid, calcium and potassium.

The food pyramid issue is best summed up by Siguel: "The beneficiaries of this policy [the pyramid] are bureaucrats protecting their jobs, researchers studying low-fat foods, corporations selling low-fat foods to an uninformed and misled public, and companies selling drugs to lower abnormal cholesterol and hypertension caused by EFA deficiency. The losers are consumers faced with increasing health-care costs, abnormal cholesterol and chronic diseases including heart disease, as well as nutritionists and patients who face conflicting and misleading guidelines."

In addition to the food imbalances promoted by the food pyramid, another problem is that it imposes general dietary guidelines for everyone, when in reality each person has very different needs.

**Build Your Own Pyramid**
The truth is that you can make your own food pyramid. Actually, that's the only sound recommendation. Since we all have individual requirements, it's best for each of us to have an individualized pyramid.

However, there are some general recommendations that may be helpful. In the following chapters we will learn that typically most people eat too much carbohydrate foods, especially refined carbohydrates. Most people also eat too much of the wrong kinds of fats and not enough of the right kinds. Many people do not get enough protein. Almost nobody eats sufficient amounts of vegetables. Worse yet, most people are deficient in the most important nutrient of all — water.

If I were to construct a food pyramid I would first make it expandable in all directions. After all, some people need more or less of certain foods and nutrients. So my adjustable pyramid would have expandable sides. It might appear tall and thin for some people and short and fat for others. But in general, my food pyramid would have some basic characteristics that make it quite different from the one promoted by the USDA.

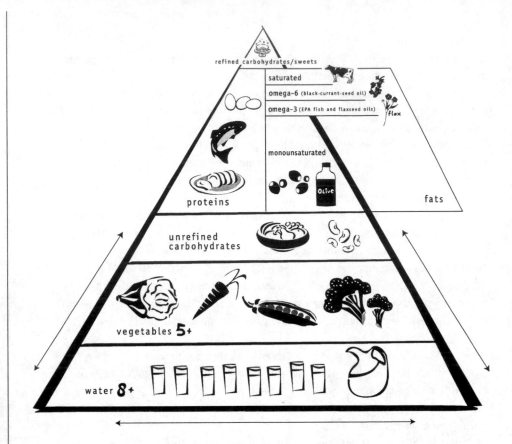

refined carbohydrates/sweets

saturated

omega-6 (black-currant-seed oil)

omega-3 (EPA fish and flaxseed oils)

flax

monounsaturated

Olive

proteins

fats

unrefined carbohydrates

vegetables **5+**

water **8+**

At the bottom of my food pyramid would be water. Water is the most important nutrient, and the one which you should consume the most of in terms of servings, volume and weight each day. Water is so important that I discuss it in its own chapter in this book.

The next layer of my food pyramid would be vegetables. I recommend eating at least five or more servings of cooked and raw vegetables daily, including a raw salad. Vegetables supply fiber, vitamins and minerals, as well as important disease-fighting phytonutrients. Vegetables are also discussed at length in a later chapter.

While carbohydrates form the base layer of the USDA's food pyramid, these types of foods would be nearer to the middle of my pyramid. And what's more they would not include refined items such as white bread and pasta, or processed cereal. Instead, my slimmer carbohydrate layer would be made up of fruits, legumes, 100-percent whole grains, and items made from 100-percent whole grains such as sprouted-grain breads.

Proteins and healthy fats would share a layer in my pyramid. Many nutritional experts are now beginning to realize that many people, including those over age 50, do not meet protein requirements. And while many people eat too much fat from saturated and omega-6 vegetable-oil sources, most people are deficient in heart-healthy monounsaturated fats such as those obtained from extra-virgin olive oil. In addition, omega-3 fats found in fish and flaxseed oil are essential and are basically devoid from the USDA pyramid. Today it is virtually impossible for people to obtain enough of these fats from a normal diet and so supplementation is often necessary.

At the top of my pyramid I would place refined carbohydrate foods such as breads, rolls and bagels made with refined flour, as well as sweets. Oddly enough, some of these items form the base of the USDA food pyramid.

In the following chapters you will be given the tools and building blocks to construct your own food pyramid. In doing so you will learn to be more intuitive about the foods that you need to achieve optimal human performance. You will learn how to find your own level of carbohydrate tolerance and your perfect balance of other macronutrients — fat and protein. Certain fats in the diet must be balanced in order for you to achieve optimal health and fitness. In addition, vegetables and fruits will become powerful allies in your quest to be fit and healthy and prevent disease. And I'll discuss the importance of the most essential nutrient of all — water. As you travel down this dietary road to better human performance, keep in mind that in all things, including diet and nutrition, balance is the key and only you can determine which balance is right for you. Choose your food wisely.

# 6 The Carbohydrate Trend

In the previous chapter we explored how the USDA food pyramid and many other contemporary diet plans stress eating large amounts of carbohydrates and minimizing protein and fat. Unfortunately, most people already consume too much carbohydrate. If you follow the USDA food pyramid recommendations, much or most of your diet is carbohydrate. For the majority of people, this can create a dietary imbalance.

One reason for this imbalance is that the human body is not adapted to processing this amount of carbohydrate, especially refined carbohydrates. For 99.6 percent of our existence on earth, humans consumed diets that averaged almost 30 percent protein with about 30 percent carbohydrates and the rest fat. During most of evolutionary history, humans lived near the sea and consumed significant amounts of fish, seafood, and other land-animal proteins. More importantly, significant amounts of plant foods were also consumed. These included vegetables, fruits, nuts and seeds, which help protect against the potential effects of high intakes of saturated fat.

In addition, early humans were very active physically. Only in the last 10,000 years has this changed. The Agricultural Revolution brought a dramatic increase in carbohydrate intake, and the Industrial Revolution brought highly refined carbohydrates to the table. The intake of carbohydrates by humans has never been so dramatically high as it has been in the last 100 years. This relatively short period of significant dietary change has contributed to many problems leading to heart disease, cancer, obesity and other diseases.

This explains why, for many people, eating carbohydrate foods can prevent a higher percentage of fats from being used for energy, lead to an increase in body-fat storage, greatly diminish human performance and negatively affect health. Yet, in the last few decades the nutritional trend has been toward a more high-carbohydrate, low-protein and low-fat diet. Many people have a strong emotional attachment to this belief, created mainly through advertising and misguided public-education campaigns.

## Carbohydrates and Insulin Production

Carbohydrate foods include breads and other items made with flour such as rolls, muffins, pancakes, waffles and pasta. Also included in this category are cereals, potatoes, and, of course, all sweets. The physiological problems associated with eating these foods have to do predominantly with insulin resistance and excess insulin production. Insulin is a hormone made by the pancreas. When you eat carbohydrate foods, they are digested and the carbohydrate is absorbed into the blood as glucose (blood sugar). This stimulates the release of insulin, which has many different jobs. Three key actions of insulin on blood sugar include the following:

- About 50 percent of the carbohydrate you eat is quickly used to fuel energy production in the body's cells. (Earlier we talked about getting energy from sugar and fat — this is the part that comes from sugar.)

- About 10 percent of the carbohydrate you eat is converted to and stored as glycogen, a reserved form of sugar. When blood sugar is low, glycogen stored in the muscles and liver is converted back to glucose for energy production. Muscle glycogen is used for energy by the muscles containing it, and liver glycogen is used mostly to maintain blood-sugar levels between meals and during nighttime sleep.

- About 40 percent of the carbohydrate you eat is converted to fat and stored.

Insulin production occurs as a normal process each and every time you eat a meal containing carbohydrates. Small amounts of insulin may also be produced if you consume a protein-only meal, and in some people, a high-protein meal can stimulate significant amounts of insulin. But for most people, it's predominantly carbohydrates that trigger the insulin mechanism.

For many people, eating carbohydrates results in production of too much insulin. For some reason or reasons not fully understood, some people have cells that become increasingly more insulin-resistant. In fact, this may have been quite normal in many of our ancestors. In people with insulin resistance, insulin can't efficiently fuel the cells, especially the muscle cells, with glucose. As a result, the cells do not get all the glucose they need to produce energy. Each time these people eat carbohydrates, the brain gets the message that the cells don't have enough sugar and the brain tells the pancreas to make more insulin. Finally, insulin is produced beyond normal limits, a condition referred to as hyperinsulinism — too much insulin. While it takes more insulin to get glucose into the insulin-resistant cells efficiently, this hormone still performs its other tasks, including converting carbohydrates to fat. As mentioned previously, in a normal person, 40 percent of the carbohydrate eaten is converted to fat. In a person who produces too much insulin, that number may be much higher, perhaps 50 to 60 percent.

In many people, this excess production of insulin may be amplified due to genetics, or it may be a normal response to eating too much carbohydrate. If you have a family history of diabetes, heart disease, high blood pressure or stroke, the odds are greater that you have less tolerance for carbohydrate consumption. Lifestyle also contributes to this problem, including poor dietary habits such as eating too much carbohydrate, too little protein and too little essential fats, lack of exercise and stress. But even if diabetes runs in your family, you still may be able to control the problem with the proper lifestyle factors.

In addition to causing even more carbohydrate to convert and store as fat, excess insulin may lower blood sugar too drastically. Since the brain relies on glucose for fuel, this can result in impaired mental function or loss of concentration. Low blood sugar also often results in hunger, sometimes only a couple of hours, or less, after the meal. Cravings, often for sweets, are frequently part of this cycle, and resorting to snacking on more carbohydrates maintains the cycle. And if you don't eat, you just feel worse. Eventually, the fat-storage deposits get bigger.

High insulin levels also suppress two important hormones: glucagon and growth hormone. Glucagon has the opposite effect of insulin and is produced following protein consumption. While insulin promotes storage, glucagon promotes the utilization of fat and sugar for energy. Growth hormone is also important for sugar- and fat-burning, the regulation of minerals, and amino-acid action on muscle development. Insulin is also important in the regulation of amino acids, the reason some insulin is secreted following a protein meal.

If your goal is to burn more body fat, improve your health and increase human performance, you must moderate carbohydrate intake by finding out how much carbohydrate your body can effectively metabolize. This will vary from person to person. Before discussing how that is accomplished, let's look at some other important aspects of carbohydrates and insulin.

**Measuring the Insulin Response**
The *glycemic index* (GI) is a very general measure of how much your blood sugar increases after eating specific carbohydrates. However, it must be noted that glycemic index is only a very general measure of individual responses to food, and individual variation is not considered in studies of foods and their glycemic

effects. High-GI foods, which produce the greatest glucose response, include bagels, breads, potatoes, sweets and other foods that contain refined flour and sugar. Some processed cereals, especially those containing the sugar maltose, produce an even stronger glucose response. Even foods you may think are good for you can trigger high amounts of insulin, including fruit juice and bananas. The three biggest problems in most diets may be wheat products, potatoes and sugar or sugar-containing products.

Carbohydrates with a lower GI include some fruits, such as grapefruits and cherries, and legumes such as lentils. Non-carbohydrate foods, proteins, and fats usually don't cause a glycemic problem, although in some people even meals high in protein and/or fat can trigger an abnormal insulin response. In these situations, eating smaller and more frequent low-glycemic meals often solves the problem, as discussed in a later chapter about healthy snacking. Most vegetables contain only small amounts of carbohydrates (except very starchy ones like potatoes and corn). Carrots were at one time believed to be a high-glycemic food, but new studies show the glycemic effect of this root vegetable to be relatively low.

Insulin responses to carbohydrate intake and the ensuing blood-sugar rise can vary greatly from person to person. But generally, more refined carbohydrates evoke a stronger and more rapid production of insulin. One reason for this, as discussed earlier, is that humans are not adapted to diets high in carbohydrate. Another reason is that refined carbohydrates lack the natural fiber that helps to moderate the carbohydrate/glucose and insulin responses. Consumption of natural fiber with carbohydrates can reduce the dietary stress associated with high-carbohydrate meals.

In practical terms, this means that eating refined foods like a cookie or piece of cake will cause more problems than eating a piece of fruit or whole-grain crackers with the same amount of carbohydrate. Low-fat foods or low-fat meals that also contain carbohydrates have a relatively higher glycemic index. This is due to quicker digestion and absorption of sugar when less fat is present. Eating carbohydrate foods in combination with some fats, such as olive oil or butter, slows digestion and absorption, thus moderating the insulin response. However, as noted previously, eating a meal very high in protein may actually increase the insulin response in some people. Artificial sweeteners should also be avoided as even these foods can cause insulin responses through what is known as the cephalic phase of digestion, in which even thinking about, seeing or tasting food causes the brain to respond by releasing insulin.

Clearly high carbohydrate intake, especially of refined carbohydrates such as bread and high-starch foods such as potatoes, is a prevalent dietary stress resulting in the overproduction of insulin and all the problems associated with it. By moderating carbohydrate intake to control your insulin production, you can increase your ability to burn fat as an optimal and efficient source of almost unlimited energy. Rather than using the glycemic index as a guide, which is common, especially among diabetics, all individuals should learn which foods and food combinations work best for their individual needs. This is most easily accomplished by performing the Two-Week Test, complete with proper follow-up, as discussed in the next chapter.

## Carbohydrate Intolerance

*Carbohydrate intolerance*, or CI, is a very common problem in many populations, and the diseases associated with this condition are reaching epidemic proportions. CI begins as a functional problem that negatively affects quality of life and which can result in serious illness and disease. Though most people are unaware such a condition even exists in its early stages, a high percentage of the population suffers from CI in its early and later stages. The symptoms of early CI are very common and include sleepiness after meals, intestinal bloating, increased body fat, fatigue and many others.

CI is called many things by many health-care professionals but it is best viewed as one long progression of the same problem. In the early stages, the symptoms include elusive problems associated with blood-sugar handling, such as fatigue, intestinal bloating and loss of concentration. In the middle stages, the problem worsens and a condition referred to as carbohydrate-lipid metabolism disturbance becomes more evident. This is the beginning of more serious conditions that include hypertension, elevations of LDL and lowering of HDL cholesterol, elevated triglycerides, excess body fat and often obesity. In the long term, CI manifests itself as various diseases, including diabetes, cancer and heart disease. These end-stage conditions are part of a set of diseases now well recognized and referred to as Syndrome X, or the Metabolic Syndrome, as discussed later in this chapter. But from beginning to end, the problem can simply be referred to as CI.

Young people with CI are at much higher risk for disease later in life. For example, those with CI have an estimated tenfold greater risk for developing diseases such as diabetes. Some individuals who ultimately become diabetic display symptoms of carbohydrate intolerance 20 years or more before the onset of disease.

Like many problems, CI is an individual one, affecting different people in different ways. Only you can determine how intolerant you are to carbohydrates, and to what degree. Blood tests will diagnose the problem only in the latter stages, but the symptoms may have begun years earlier. The key to avoiding disease is to be aware of CI in its earliest stage, and to make the appropriate diet and lifestyle changes. This will improve quality of life immediately and prevent the onset of disease later. However, for those already in a disease state, significant immediate improvements in quality of life can still be made with the proper adjustments. It's up to you to find your body's limit of carbohydrate foods and determine how much of these foods is excessive. It's easy to do, and I'll discuss how it's done in the following chapter.

Following is a list of some common complaints of people with CI. Many symptoms occur immediately following a meal that contains carbohydrates, and others are constant. While keeping in mind that these symptoms may also be related to other causes, ask yourself if you have any of these problems:

- **Physical fatigue.** Whether you call it fatigue or exhaustion, the most common feature of CI is that it wears people out. Some are tired just in the morning or afternoon; others are exhausted all day.

- **Mental fatigue.** Sometimes the fatigue of CI is physical, but often it's mental (as opposed to psychological); the inability to concentrate is the most evident symptom. Loss of creativity, poor memory, and failing or poor grades in school often accompany CI, as do various forms of "learning disabilities." This is much more pronounced immediately after a meal, or if a meal is delayed or missed. The worker who returns to his or her job site after lunch, only to be unable to concentrate due to mental fatigue, is a very common example.

- **Blood-sugar handling problems.** Fluctuations in blood sugar are normal during the day, but may be amplified if meals are not eaten on a regular schedule. Periods of erratic blood sugar, including abnormal hypoglycemia, accompanied by many of the symptoms listed here, are not normal. Feeling jittery, agitated and moody is common with CI, and is relieved almost immediately once food is eaten. Dizziness is also common, as is the craving for sweets, chocolate or caffeine. These bouts occur more frequently between meals or if meals are not eaten on time. These symptoms are not necessarily associated with abnormal blood-sugar levels, but may be related to neurological stress, possibly due to the changes in blood sugar and insulin.

☐ **Intestinal bloating.** Most intestinal gas is produced from dietary carbohydrates, specifically the high-starch types such as wheat and potatoes. People with CI who eat carbohydrates suffer from excessive gas production. Antacids, or other remedies for symptomatic relief, are not very successful in dealing with the problem. The gas tends to build and is worse later in the day and at night.

☐ **Sleepiness.** Many people with CI get sleepy immediately after meals containing more than their limit of carbohydrates. This is typically a pasta meal, or even a meat meal that includes bread, potatoes or dessert.

☐ **Increased fat storage and weight.** For most people, too much weight is too much fat. In males, an increase in abdominal fat is more evident and an early sign of CI (I call this the "carbo belly"). In females, it's more prominent in the upper body compared to the thighs and legs. In the face, "chipmunk cheeks" may be a telltale sign.

☐ **Increased triglycerides.** High triglycerides in the blood are often seen in overweight people. But even those who are not fat may have stores of fat in their arteries as a result of CI. These triglycerides are the direct result of carbohydrates from the diet being converted by insulin into fat. In my experience, fasting triglyceride levels over 100 mg/dl may be an indication of a carbohydrate-intolerance problem, even though 100 is in the so-called normal range.

☐ **Increased blood pressure.** It is well known that many if not most people with hypertension produce too much insulin and are carbohydrate-intolerant. It is often possible to show a direct relationship between insulin levels and blood pressure

— as insulin levels elevate, so does blood pressure. For some, regardless of whether the blood pressure is elevated, sodium sensitivity is common and eating too much sodium causes water retention along with elevated blood pressure.

☑ **Depression.** Because carbohydrates can be a natural "downer," depression is common among people who have CI. Carbohydrates do this by adversely affecting levels of neurotransmitters made in the brain. This may produce a feeling of depression or sleepiness. Many people have been taught that sugar is stimulating, but actually the opposite can be true. This is a significant consideration for children or adults trying to function optimally at school, home or work.

☑ **Addiction.** CI is also prevalent in persons addicted to alcohol, caffeine, cigarettes or other drugs. Often, the drug is the secondary problem, with CI being the primary one. Treating this primary problem should obviously be a major focus of any addiction therapy.

In addition to people who eat too many carbohydrates, those most vulnerable for carbohydrate intolerance include people who are inactive, under stress, or taking estrogen, and those with a family history of diabetes. In addition, aging is frequently accompanied by increased carbohydrate intolerance.

When a person with this problem lowers carbohydrate intake to tolerable levels, many, if not most, of the other symptoms may disappear. With the stress of CI eliminated, the body is finally able to correct many of its own problems.

**Syndrome X**

If the problems mentioned above are not corrected, your symptoms and your health can get much worse. If CI persists, this functional problem can lead to disease, specifically a whole complex of related diseases that include some of the biggest killers of today: heart disease, cancer, stroke and diabetes. These diseases kill more people in the United States each year than died in all of our wars combined. As CI progresses it can lead to an entire complex of diseases referred to as Syndrome X. The specific disorders include:

- Hyperinsulinemia

- Diabetes (type 2)

- Hypertension

- Obesity

- Polycystic ovary

- Stroke

- Breast cancer

- Coronary heart disease

- Hyperlipidemia (high blood cholesterol and triglycerides)

These problems don't necessarily all develop or even evolve in this order. But all are related to CI. Unfortunately, once some of these diseases develop, many of the changes are permanent and more radical care is needed. However, even these conditions can improve with the right dietary control, which includes solving the problem of excess carbohydrate intake (along with getting adequate exercise).

How do you adjust your lifestyle so that carbohydrate intolerance is not a problem? Before you do anything, you need to know just how sensitive, if at all, you are to dietary carbohydrates. Your doctor may do some tests, including checking insulin and glucose levels, to see if the problem can be detected. You could just follow a low-carbohydrate diet, but the better choice is to determine just what your own specific needs are, and modify them as the years go by.

Finding your optimal level of carbohydrate intake is the first step to balancing the rest of your diet. For many years I have been using an effective method of finding the optimal level of carbohydrate intake. It's called the Two-Week Test and is detailed in the following chapter.

# 7 The Two-Week Test

The Two-Week Test described in this chapter will provide you with vital information to help you determine if you have carbohydrate intolerance, and if you do, it will get you on the right track to determining your optimal level of carbohydrate intake. First let me stress that this is only a test, and it will only last two weeks. You will not be eating like this forever.

The Two-Week Test provides you with a period of time in which your insulin levels remain relatively low because your carbohydrate intake is decreased. Before you start the test, ask yourself about the signs and symptoms of carbohydrate intolerance described in the previous chapter. Write down the problems that you have from this list, along with any other complaints you have. After the test, you will ask yourself again how you feel regarding these complaints. In addition, if you are concerned about your weight, weigh yourself before starting the test. This is the only instance I recommend using the scale.

Before you start the test, make sure you have enough of the foods you'll be eating during the test. Go shopping and stock up on these items. In addition, go through your cabinets and refrigerator and get rid of any sweets in your house, or you'll be tempted.

Do not go hungry during the test! There are many foods to select from so you don't ever need to go hungry. Eat as many eggs as you want, as much cheese or meat, and as many vegetables as you need to feel full. Don't worry about cholesterol, fat or calories, or the amount of food you're eating. This is balanced in the next steps.

The test should not be difficult, although it is probably a big change from the way you were eating previously. Many individuals with CI have been on a high-carbohydrate, low-fat and low-protein diet. If you've been eating lots of sweets or other carbohydrates, you may experience cravings for sugar for a few days during the test. Some have referred to this as a carbohydrate addiction. If you get such cravings, eat something on the acceptable list instead and stick it out.

Following the test for less than two weeks probably will not yield valid results. So if after five days you eat a bowl of pasta you'll need to start over.

Avoid all anaerobic exercise, including weight-lifting and other more-strenuous activities, during the test (see exercise section later in this book).

As for the test itself, you merely want to eat using the following guidelines for a period of no less than two weeks.

### Foods to Avoid

You may not eat any of the following foods during the Two-Week Test:

- Bread, rolls, pasta, pancakes, cereal, muffins, chips, crackers and rice cakes.
- Sweets, including products that contain sugar such as ketchup, honey, and many other prepared foods (read the labels).
- Fruits and fruit juice.
- Highly processed meats such as cold cuts, which often contain sugar.
- Potatoes (all types), corn, rice and beans.
- Milk, half-and-half and yogurt.
- So-called healthy snacks, including all energy bars and drinks.
- All soda, including diet, and alcohol, except small amounts of dry wine.

### Foods to Eat

You may eat as much of the following foods as you like during the Two-Week Test:

- Whole eggs, unprocessed, fully cultured cheeses, cream.
- Unprocessed meats including beef, turkey, chicken, lamb, fish, shellfish and others.
- Tomato, V-8 or other vegetable juices such as carrot juice.
- Cooked or raw vegetables except potatoes and corn.
- Nuts, seeds, nut butters.
- Oils, vinegar, mayonnaise, salsa and mustard (read the label to make sure there are no added sugars or hydrogenated oils).
- Sea salt, unless you are sodium sensitive.
- Water! During the Two-Week Test and forever after, be sure to drink plenty of water. Most people need at least six to ten 8-ounce glasses of water per day. Generally, the more protein you consume, the more water you will need between meals.

### Helpful Suggestions

Following are some other suggestions for eating, food preparation and dining out which may be helpful during the Two-Week Test. You may find these suggestions helpful after completing the test as well.

### Meal Ideas

*Eggs*
- Omelets, with any combination of vegetables, meats and cheeses.
- Scrambled with guacamole, sour cream and salsa.
- Scrambled with a scoop of ricotta or cottage cheese and tomato sauce.

- Boiled or poached with spinach or asparagus and hollandaise or cheese sauce.
- Add turkey or chicken slices if appealing.
- Soufflés.

### Salads
- Chef — leaf lettuce, meats, cheeses, eggs.
- Spinach — with bacon, eggs, anchovies.
- Caesar — Romaine lettuce, eggs, Parmesan cheese, anchovies.
- Any salad with chicken, tuna, shrimp or other meat or cheese.

### Salad Dressings
- Extra-virgin olive oil and vinegar (balsamic, wine, apple cider). Plain or with sea salt and spices.
- Creamy — made with heavy cream, mayonnaise, garlic and spices.

### Fish and Meats
- Pot roast cooked with onions, carrots and celery.
- Roasted chicken stuffed with a bulb of anise, celery and carrots.
- Chili made with fresh, chopped meat and a variety of vegetables such as diced eggplant, onions, celery, peppers, zucchini, tomatoes and spices.
- Steak and eggs.
- Any meat with a vegetable and a mixed salad.
- Chicken parmigiana (not breaded or deep-fried) with a mixed salad.
- Fish (not breaded or fried) with any variety of sauces and vegetables.
- Tuna melt on a bed of broccoli or asparagus.

### Sauces
- A quick cream sauce can be made by simmering heavy cream with mustard or curry powder and cayenne pepper, or any flavor of choice. It's delicious over eggs, poultry and vegetables.
- Italian-style tomato sauce helps makes a quick parmigiana out of any fish, meat or vegetables. Put this over spaghetti squash for a vegetarian pasta-like dish. Or make a "lasagna" out of slices of eggplant or zucchini instead of pasta.

### Snacks
- Celery stuffed with nut butter or cream cheese.
- Guacamole with vegetable sticks for dipping.
- Hard-boiled eggs.

- Rolled slices of fresh meat and cheese.
- Vegetable juices.
- Almonds, cashews, pecans, sunflower seeds.

### Dining Out
- Let the waiter know you do not want any bread, to avoid temptation.
- Don't hesitate to ask for an extra vegetable instead of rice or potato.
- Avoid all fried food.
- Avoid iceberg lettuce. Choose a Caesar or spinach salad instead.

### Dining Menu Options
- Chinese: Steamed dishes or moo shu (no rice, pancakes or sweet sauce).
- Continental: Filet mignon or other steak, duck, fish or seafood.
- French: Coquille Saint-Jacques, boeuf a la Bourguignonne.
- Italian: Veal parmigiana (not breaded or deep-fried), mussels marinara.
- Vegetarian: Tofu or cheese and vegetables, egg dishes.

### Evaluating the Results
After the Two-Week Test, re-evaluate your list of complaints. If nothing improved, then you may not be carbohydrate intolerant. But if you feel better now than you did two weeks ago, or if you lost weight, chances are you may have some degree of CI. Some people who have a high degree of CI will feel much better than they did before the test, especially if there was a large weight loss. Some people say they feel like a new person after taking this test.

Any weight loss during the test is not due to reduced calories, as many people eat more calories than usual during this two-week period. It's due to the increased fat-burning resulting from reduced insulin. While there may be some water loss, especially if you are sodium sensitive, there is real fat loss.

If your blood pressure has been high, and especially if you are on medication, ask your health-care professional to check it several times during the test. Sometimes blood pressure drops significantly and your medication may need to be adjusted, which should only be done upon recommendation of your health-care professional.

### Finding Your Carbohydrate Tolerance
If the Two-Week Test improved your signs and symptoms, the next step is to determine how much carbohydrate you can tolerate, without a return of these problems. This is done in the following manner.

Begin adding small amounts of carbohydrates to your diet with every other meal or snack. This may be a slice of bread at lunch, or a half of potato with dinner. Whatever you add, make sure it's not a refined carbohydrate: no foods containing sugar, no refined-flour products (like white bread, rolls or pasta), brown rice instead of white, etc. Don't add a carbohydrate to back-to-back meals, as insulin production is partly influenced by your previous meal.

With each addition of carbohydrate, watch for any of the symptoms you had previously that were eliminated by the test. Look especially for symptoms that develop immediately after eating, such as intestinal bloating, sleepiness or feelings of depression. If your hunger or cravings disappeared during the two weeks and now have returned, you've probably eaten too many carbohydrates. If you lost 8 pounds during the test, and gained back 5 pounds after adding some carbohydrates for a week or two, you've probably eaten too many carbohydrates.

## Reality Check

Once you've found your body's ideal level of carbohydrate intake, it will be relatively easy to maintain your intake. You'll be able to eat almost anything you want once you know your limit. And you probably won't want to eat more than your limit because you'll become acutely aware of how bad your body feels when you eat too many carbohydrates. From time to time, you may feel the need to go through a Two-Week Test period to check yourself and make sure your tolerance has not changed, or to get back on track after careless eating during the holidays, vacations or at other times.

Many people find the loss of grains in the diet leaves the digestive tract sluggish, which may make you a little constipated. If you become constipated during the Two-Week Test, or afterwards when a lower amount of carbohydrate in the diet is maintained, it could be due to any or all of three reasons. First, you may not be eating enough fiber. Bread, pasta and cereals are significant sources of fiber for many people. But so are vegetables and legumes, such as lentils, which are low-glycemic. So if you become constipated, it may simply be that you need to eat more vegetables. And once you learn how much carbohydrate you can tolerate in your diet, adding that will also help, especially if you can tolerate some fruit. Adding plain unsweetened psyllium (available in health-food stores) to a glass of water or tomato juice will keep your system running smoothly. Another way to add psyllium to your diet is to use it in place of flour for thickening sauces or in place of bread crumbs to coat meats and vegetables. If you require a fiber supplement, be sure to use the ones that do not contain sugar. Most fiber products contain sugar, so read the labels. There are many sugar-free psyllium products on the market so you should not have trouble finding one. One teaspoon per day is usually enough to maintain regularity.

**A Note about Ketosis**

When your body starts using more fats for energy, as is the case during the Two-Week Test, the liver produces three substances collectively called ketone bodies. When levels of ketone bodies are higher than about 1 mg/dl, the condition is referred to as ketosis. Only in extreme states will this normal state of ketosis turn into an abnormal condition called ketoacidosis, in which the body has become too acid due to the loss of alkaline reserve.

When you severly limit carbohydrate intake, your body may not completely burn all the ketone bodies produced. Another way of explaining it is that you are burning much more fat than you can use for energy. The result is that some fat is not completely burned and ends up being ketone bodies. These are eliminated in the urine and stools, and also by breath via the lungs.

Some of these ketone bodies are also used as fuel by many parts of the body, including the brain and heart. Any level of ketosis can be measured by a simple blood test, or by testing urine with ketone sticks, available in drug stores. I do not recommend focusing on ketone-body production as some diet programs do. I don't feel it is necessary to get into a state of ketosis in order to be successful. In measuring patients following the Two-Week Test, I have found that some produce excess ketone bodies and others don't, regardless of their success with signs and symptoms.

Another reason for constipation at this time may be dehydration. If you don't drink enough water, you could be predisposed to constipation. During the Two-Week Test, you'll need more water — up to three quarts or more per day. For some people, drinking gallons of water still won't prevent constipation. This could be due to eicosanoid imbalance which is discussed in later chapters on dietary fats. For now, just remember that if more water does not help a possible reason for constipation is there is not enough oil in the diet.

Occasionally, some people will get very tired during the Two-Week Test. This can be due to a number of problems. Ask yourself:

- Am I drinking enough water?

- Am I eating enough food?

- Am I eating as often as necessary (i.e., sometimes every two or three hours)?

• Am I eating carbohydrates without realizing it?

• If I am not sodium sensitive, am I getting enough salt?

• Am I eating enough vegetables?

### Case History

*Bob was determined to renew his health in a natural way. He was overweight and overfat, always exhausted, and his blood pressure, cholesterol and triglycerides were too high. He took the Two-Week Test and initially felt very good. But within a few days he began getting tired and irritable. After talking with Bob for just a few minutes, it was clear that he was doing several things wrong. Because it caused him to spend more time in bathrooms, he did not drink much water during the day. In addition, since he thought about how many calories he was eating he became calorie conscious and ate less. To make matters worse, he thought that yogurt was in the cheese group, and was eating two or three containers of fruit yogurt each day. When I told Bob that the yogurt had 6 to 7 teaspoons of sugar in each container, and to forget about the calories for now and force the water, he started his test again. After the first week he was feeling great. Within a month, his energy was being maintained, blood pressure and blood fats were back to normal, and he lost 14 pounds.*

### Maintaining Your Balance

Once you successfully finish the Two-Week Test, and add back the right amount of carbohydrates to your diet, you should have a very good idea of your carbohydrate limits. This is best accomplished by asking yourself about your signs and symptoms on a regular basis: energy, weight, sleepiness and bloating after meals, etc. You may want to keep a diary so you can be more objective in your self-assessment. In time, you won't need to focus as much on this issue as your intuition will take over and you'll automatically know your limits.

If you need help in going from the calorie/gram/percentage-counting game to being intuitive, you can sneak a peek at the carbohydrate levels of foods by looking at food labels. But realize that the amount of carbohydrate in food has two components: one is the part that you absorb and becomes blood glucose, which increases insulin. The other part is the fiber portion, which is not absorbed. So when calculating the carbohydrate content of a food or meal, remember to subtract the grams of fiber from the total grams of carbohydrate to get the actual amount that will affect your metabolism. This is easy to do; look at the food label found on all packaged items. Read the amount of total carbohydrate, then subtract the amount of fiber. This will equal your usable carbohydrate. This is another reason counting calories, grams or percentages of macronutrients can be very misleading.

Once you find your level of tolerance — the amount of carbohydrate you can eat without producing symptoms — you can easily relate that amount to grams or calories of carbohydrates. Most diets have you start with that number, and suggest that you don't exceed a specified number. But ideally, you want to know your limit by experience and intuition. It's not hard to do.

Once you find your level of carbohydrate tolerance, you're on your way to balancing your whole diet. Remember, don't be afraid to eat at your level of tolerance for carbohydrates, even if people tell you you're crazy. Now that you know how much carbohydrate you can tolerate, in the next chapter I'll discuss which types of carbohydrate foods are the healthiest to eat.

# 8 Carbohydrates: The Good and the Bad

After you determine the amount of carbohydrate you can tolerate it's likely that these types of foods will remain a substantial percentage of your diet, typically up to 40 percent. When choosing carbohydrate foods it's important to realize that not all are created equal. Some carbohydrates are more natural than others, thus the response they evoke in the body is less dramatic. In general, the more highly processed the carbohydrate food, the worse it is for you. Highly processed carbohydrates generally have a higher glycemic index than those that are processed less or not processed at all. This is true of most commercially processed bread, bagels, rolls, cereals and other foods. These foods should be avoided or at the very least minimized. Some carbohydrate foods — such as most desserts and sweets — are so highly processed that they have virtually no nutritional value. Once your body is balanced you should be able to occasionally consume some sugar, a small dessert or other junk food without ill effects. Until then, it's best to carefully assess the type of carbohydrate foods that you eat and choose the healthiest items possible.

So what carbohydrates should you eat? At the top of the list of unprocessed carbohydrates is fruit. In addition to containing vitamins and minerals, fruit also contains important phytonutrients. Though fruit is a carbohydrate food, the glycemic index of most fruit is low to moderate because fruit contains substantial amounts of fiber, and because fruit sugar, or fructose, has the lowest glycemic index of all sugars. Most fruits contain a combination of fructose and glucose, and those with the most fructose have a lower glycemic index. At the low end of the glycemic index are cherries, plums, grapefruits, apricots and peaches. Apples and pears have a more moderate glycemic index, with grapes, oranges and bananas scoring higher. Pineapple and watermelon are among the highest-glycemic fruits and should be eaten sparingly.

Legumes or beans are thought by many to be a protein food. But the truth is most legumes contain much more carbohydrate than protein. For instance a serving of red beans typically may have 6 grams of protein and 16 grams of carbohydrate, with 5 of these carbohydrate grams as fiber. As mentioned previously, if you read labels you should subtract the fiber from the carbohydrate total to get the actual usable carbohydrate content. So you can see that even after subtracting the fiber, red beans contain nearly twice as much starch, or sugar, as protein. However, because of the presence of both protein and fiber, the glycemic index of red beans and other legumes remains relatively low for a carbohydrate food. In addition, other legumes may have even lower glycemic effects. Peanuts, for example, have a very low glycemic index because they are not only low in carbohydrate but also high in fat. Soybeans also have a low GI due to their high content of both protein and fiber. Overall, because of their composition, most beans, including lentils, have a moderate glycemic effect, and are a good alternative to refined-carbohydrate foods.

Many people consume the bulk of their carbohydrates as grains. Whole grains, and products made from them, are more healthful than their refined counterparts, containing more of the nutrients and fiber from the original grain. For instance, whole oat groats are better than oatmeal, and regular oatmeal is better than "quick" oats. Long-grain brown rice is better than short-grain white rice. Wild rice, which isn't really a rice but a seed from a reedy grass, is fairly low in carbohydrate and has a moderate glycemic index as well. If you choose to eat bread or pasta, it's best to find 100-percent whole-grain products rather than those made from refined flour. In addition there are a number of breads on the market made from whole, sprouted grains. Processed wheat flour (white flour) can increase insulin levels two to three times more than true whole-grain products.

Vegetables can also be a significant source of carbohydrates, though most contain only small amounts. Vegetables are an extremely important item in the diet and are discussed in detail later in this section. Some vegetables, however, contain moderate to high amounts of carbohydrates and therefore warrant discussion here. Among the higher-carbohydrate vegetables are corn and potatoes, which should be eaten sparingly. In fact, a baked potato has a whopping 37 grams of carbohydrate — as much as a serving of cooked pasta — and a higher glycemic index than some cakes and candy. New potatoes have a much lower glycemic index than other varieties.

**Wheat: The Shaft of Life?**
One grain to be very careful about eating is wheat. Over the centuries, wheat has become the staple of many diets. This is very unfortunate, as wheat is a common cause of intestinal problems, allergies and sometimes disease. Wheat also can prevent absorption of various nutrients, induce weight gain and trigger other health problems.

Some people are more sensitive to the harmful effects of wheat than others. The most practical way to tell is to note how you feel after eating wheat or products made from it, such as pasta, bread, bagels, cereal and most snack foods, such as cookies and pretzels. The most common symptom is intestinal bloating, but may also include belching, diarrhea or other abdominal discomfort, as well as reduced mental focus or sleepiness.

Wheat can bind important minerals such as calcium, magnesium, iron, zinc and copper from food and prevent their absorption. This grain can also reduce digestive enzymes, especially those from the pancreas, rendering key foods — including protein and fats — less digestible. With this reduced protein digestion, whole proteins could be absorbed, which could lead to allergies. With poor fat digestion, essential fatty acids may not be absorbed, leading to problems such as reduced skin quality, inflammation and hormonal imbalance. Eating wheat and then exercising can trigger allergic reactions in some people. These reactions range from mild problems, like skin rash or hives, to more severe problems including anaphylaxis and occasionally even death.

If you're sensitive to wheat, reducing or eliminating it from your diet is the most effective way to correct the problem and reduce the unhealthy effects.

## What about Sweeteners?

Sweeteners are carbohydrates, or sugars, in their purest form. They range from highly processed and high-glycemic products such as maltodextrin, to the relatively moderate sucrose and honey, to pure fructose, which has the lowest glycemic index of all sugars. As with other carbohydrate foods, the least processed and more natural sugars are best to use if you need a sweetener.

Honey has been used for centuries as both a sweetener and a remedy, and remains today as the most natural sweetener available. Honey contains a variety of vitamins, minerals and amino acids, including antioxidants. In addition, honey has anti-inflammatory and antimicrobial effects. Recently a large volume of scientific literature has substantiated honey's therapeutic value, as well as its ability to improve endurance in athletes.

Honey is also perhaps the only carbohydrate food that does not promote tooth decay through acidity. In general, proteins and fats raise salivary pH, making it more alkaline, while carbohydrate foods lower pH, making it more acidic. Honey is the sweet exception — a carbohydrate that may raise pH levels. In addition, honey has an overall beneficial effect on oral health due to its antibacterial effect and ability to reduce dextran, a sticky, sugary substance that helps bacteria adhere to the teeth.

Like fruit, honey is primarily a blend of fructose and glucose, typically about 38 and 31 percent respectively. Different types of honey have different ratios of each type of sugar. Those which crystallize the fastest are the ones with the highest glucose content, and thus the higher glycemic index. Since fructose has the lowest glycemic index of all sugars, honey with higher fructose content will have the lowest glycemic index. Sage honey, for example is known for its high fructose content, while clover honey has a medium fructose content, and alfalfa honey is higher in glucose.

When shopping for honey, look for a number of attributes. Dark honey may be the most therapeutic and have the most nutrients. Buckwheat honey is said to contain the highest amounts of antioxidants. Raw, unfiltered honey retains more beneficial qualities. Heat, light and filtering remove some of the beneficial properties of honey.

### What about Artificial Sweeteners?

Do you really think you're saving calories by choosing an artificial sugar substitute over the real thing? There are two main issues regarding the use of fake sugars — what they do to your metabolism, and how they affect your health.

The argument that artificial sweeteners may have harmful dietary effects on health is still raging. Substances such as saccharin are not recommended for children or pregnant women, and aspartame has been related to an increased incidence of migraine headaches and allergic reactions. While these are important concerns, one fact has been ignored: The use of artificial sweeteners is most often accompanied by increased consumption of food. In other words, if you use artificial sweeteners, studies show you often end up eating more food, usually sweets. What's worse is that you may store more fat as well.

Researchers are unclear why this happens, but certain factors seem to be implicated. It may be a learned process by the body. The tasting of sweet substances may cause the body to store, rather than burn, fat. Or, it may be related to the dehydration that accompanies consumption of artificial sweeteners. This may trigger the brain to increase the appetite and food intake as a means of restoring water balance. Eating low-calorie substances will lower the body's metabolism. This will not only cause the body to store more fat but also activate the need to eat more food.

Artificial sweeteners are used in diet soda, chewing gum, ice cream, iced-tea mixes and many other products. If you want to avoid artificial sweeteners, you must read labels. You may be fooled into believing that you are buying a more-healthful, low-calorie food when you choose a product made with fake sugar. You're avoiding only 15 calories from a teaspoon of table sugar or honey, when using an artificial sweetener containing 1 or 2 calories. Is it worth it? That 14 or 15 extra calories is not significant for most people (although it is for those who are insulin-resistant or diabetic). These factors do not occur with regular or natural sugar. People generally eat less food, for example, when they consume sugared drinks. There are, however, many other problems associated with the intake of excess sugar. The best situation is to eliminate your addiction to sugar; Americans eat 125 pounds per person per year.

Clearly if you want to be healthy, you not only need to know your limit when it comes to carbohydrates, you also need to carefully choose what types of carbohydrates are best for you. In general, refined carbohydrates should be minimized and fake sugars avoided altogether. You'll want to choose mostly from fruits, legumes and whole grains, and use small amounts of honey as your main sweetener. As you begin to choose your carbohydrate foods more wisely, you will notice that you feel better. This is part of becoming more intuitive about your diet and individual needs. In addition to making wise choices about carbohydrate foods, you need to do the same when it comes to eating fat, which is discussed in the following chapters.

# 9  The Big Fat Lie

If you think all fats are bad for you, think again. That's a big fat lie. Fat is one of the most beneficial substances in your diet, and is often the missing ingredient in developing and maintaining good health and fitness. But a misunderstanding of the role of fats and a well-financed misinformation campaign has misled the public and led to an epidemic of fat phobia. Just think of the billions of dollars spent each year on low-fat and fat-free foods and you'll understand why you might not have been told the whole truth about fat. Does this sound astonishing? Read on.

First, let's define fat. I'm talking about vegetable oils, butter, the fats in eggs, meats and cheeses, and other naturally occurring fats. Make no mistake, these high-energy foods can be harmful if overeaten. Too much or too little is dangerous. It's simply a question of balancing your intake.

There are two factors which can disturb the delicate balance of fats. The first is eating too many of one type of fat, such as too much saturated fat from dairy products or too much omega-6 fat from vegetable oil. As we'll see, consuming balanced amounts of the different types of healthy fats can help maintain health and prevent disease. But eating processed fats, such as hydrogenated oils, and overheated fats, such as in fried foods, causes dysfunction and can lead to disease. This means some popular foods are out: chips, French fries and fried chicken, to name just a few. They're loaded with the wrong kinds of fat.

Dietary fats have been a staple for humans throughout evolution. Ironically many people are learning of the true importance of fats in the diet only since the low-fat trend of the last few decades. This is not news, really. Scientists have known of the importance of fat in the diet since the discoveries in 1929 by researchers who demonstrated the necessity of dietary fat and its many healthy functions. Here are some of them.

## Disease Prevention and Treatment

Dietary fat has been blamed for almost every disease known to mankind. However, this is a gross oversimplification of a very complicated problem. Since the public rarely gets the full story on health issues, most people have a misguided view of the connection between eating fat and developing diseases such as cancer. The truth is that certain dietary fats consumed in balanced proportions can actually help prevent many dangerous diseases. For instance, we now know that dietary fats are central to the eicosanoid system which controls inflammation.

Chronic inflammation has been linked by scientists to many of our most feared diseases. This is discussed in the following chapter, and in the last section on self-health management.

But fat may not only be instrumental in *preventing* disease, it may have a role in *treating* disease and other illness as well. Selectively increasing dietary fat has been shown to reduce the growth or spreading of malignant tumors. This is according to an article entitled "Effects of Lipids on Cancer Therapy," published in the June 1990 issue of *Nutrition Reviews*. The authors, C. Patrick Burns, M.D., and Arthur Spector, M.D., both from the University of Iowa College of Medicine, discuss how dietary fats help change cancer cell membranes and increase the production of eicosanoids. These changes greatly enhance the effectiveness of certain therapies for treating tumors and other abnormal tissue growth. In some cancers, such as mammary carcinomas, the increased intake of omega-3 fats alone had a positive therapeutic effect.

## Energy

The aerobic system depends on fats as the fuel for the aerobic muscles, which power us through the day. Fat produces energy, and prevents excessive dependency upon sugar, especially blood sugar. Fats provide more than twice as much potential energy as carbohydrates do, 9 calories per gram as opposed to only 4 calories. Your body is capable of obtaining most of its energy from fat, up to 80 or 90 percent, if your fat-burning mechanism is working efficiently. The body even uses fat as a source of energy for heart-muscle function. These fats — called phospholipids — normally are contained in the heart muscle and generate energy to make it work more efficiently.

What happens, though, if you are not able to use fat for energy? What if you have not programmed your body to burn fat? Then you must use more sugar for energy. This can create the mood swings people with blood-sugar variations often feel, especially when blood sugar gets too low. Other symptoms include mental or physical fatigue, clumsiness, headaches, psychoses, depression, allergies and other physical and mental impairments, depending on your susceptibility to an excess or deprivation of sugar in the blood.

How can you avoid these highs and lows? By making sure you burn enough fat for energy. If your body is burning fat for energy while you exercise or cook dinner or watch TV, your brain and nervous system will have enough sugar, which they require for energy. Clearly, if the rest of the body takes too much of the brain's energy supply of sugar, the brain will not function at peak performance, and neither will the rest of your body.

A second reaction to the body's not having enough balanced fat for energy is that it will store fat. Remember, the body likes fat — just think of all the foods with a high fat content that you like to eat. Actually, the body likes fat so much that carbohydrates and proteins can be converted and stored as fat. In fact, the body stores fat for the future, just in case that fat will be needed later — tomorrow, next week or next month. Let's look at some more of the various body functions that require fat.

### The Hormonal System

The hormonal system is responsible for controlling virtually all healthy functions of the body. But for this system to function properly, the body must produce proper amounts of the appropriate hormones. Many glands, such as the adrenal glands, are dependent on fat for production of hormones.

In addition to the adrenal glands, the thymus, thyroid, kidneys and other glands use fats to help make hormones. The adrenals also require a specific fat, cholesterol, for the production of hormones such as progesterone and cortisone. The thymus gland regulates immunity and the body's defense systems. The thyroid regulates temperature, weight and other metabolic functions. The kidney's hormones help regulate blood pressure, circulation and filtering of blood.

Today, many people are rightly concerned about the fat content of their bodies. But hormonal problems, and the health problems that stem from them, can be seen in those who have fat imbalances or whose body fat is too low. For example, some women who exercise too much experience disruptions in their menstrual cycle, usually indicating a fat-metabolism disorder. Many women also accept the popular misconception that menopause is always accompanied by significant complaints. In reality, women with properly functioning hormonal systems should have only minor symptoms. Many women who are on a low-fat diet, or who have a history of following a low-fat diet and have not corrected fatty-acid imbalances or deficiencies, experience significant menopausal complaints. These often are related to fatty-acid deficiencies. Without the right balance of fats in the system, the hormonal system can't produce certain hormones.

### Eicosanoid Balance

Hormone-like substances called eicosanoids are necessary for such normal cellular function as regulating inflammation, hydration, circulation and free-radical activity. Produced from dietary fats, eicosanoids are especially important for their role in controlling inflammation — the precursor of many chronic diseases including cancer, heart disease and Alzheimer's. Many people who have inflammatory conditions, such as arthritis, colitis, tendinitis — conditions whose names end in "itis" — probably have an eicosanoid imbalance. But in many more people, chronic inflammation goes on silently.

The balance of eicosanoids is also important for regulating blood pressure and hydration. An imbalance can produce high or low blood pressure, or trigger constipation or diarrhea. Eicosanoid imbalance may also be associated with menstrual cramps, blood clotting, tumor growth and other problems. The role of fat in balancing eicosanoids is discussed in detail in the following chapter.

## Insulation

The body's ability to store fat permits humans to live in most climates, especially in areas of extreme heat or cold. In warmer areas of the world, stored fat provides protection from the heat. In colder lands, increased fat stored beneath the skin prevents too much heat from leaving the body. An example of fat's effectiveness as an insulator is in the Eskimo's ability to withstand great cold and survive in good health. Eskimos eat a good deal of omega-3 fat and much of it is stored under their skin. Moreover, despite a diet heavy in these fats, Eskimos have a very low incidence of heart disease and other ailments.

In warmer climates, fat prevents too much water from leaving the body, which can result in dehydration that causes dry, scaly skin. Some evaporation is normal, of course, but fats under the skin regulate evaporation and can prevent as much as 10 to 20 times more water from leaving the body.

## Healthy Skin and Hair

It's the protective qualities of fat that give skin the soft, smooth and unwrinkled appearance that so many people try to achieve through expensive skin conditioners. The healthy look of skin comes from the fat inside. The same is true for your hair. Fats, including cholesterol, also serve as an insulating barrier within the skin. Without this protection, water and water-soluble substances such as chemical pollutants would enter the body through the skin. With the proper balance and amounts of fats in your diet, your skin and hair develop a healthy appearance. In fact, if you've been looking for the ideal skin and hair product, you can end your search by balancing the fats in your diet.

## Pregnancy and Lactation

For many years doctors told women not to gain too much weight during pregnancy; 20 to 25 pounds was the maximum weight gain advised. Many women followed this advice by eliminating fats from their diets, which created nutritional deficiencies and problems with fat metabolism. This was unhealthy for both mother and baby.

Today, more doctors are recommending higher average weight gains during pregnancy. Depending on the woman's frame and health, up to 30 or more pounds is acceptable. This has been shown to result in healthier babies and mothers, so long as the mother is active in the months after birth.

The time to improve your health is long before you decide to have a baby. Being in a state of good health will make conceiving a child much easier. This applies to males as well as females. The effective functioning of the hormonal system is important to both would-be parents. Once conception does take place, fats are important to the continued good health of the mother and child.

The uterus must maintain the health of the newly conceived embryo by providing nutrition until the placenta can begin to function, usually a period of a week or more. If there is an adequate level of progesterone, which is produced from fats, there should be enough nutrients for the newly-formed embryo to survive the first critical week. Without enough progesterone, the embryo could die.

In addition, the placenta must form and be in good functioning order, producing hormones that affect the developing fetus. Both of these hormones — estrogen and progesterone — are fat-dependent and are produced in increasing quantities as the pregnancy continues. Together they promote the growth of the uterus and the storage of nutrients for the fetus. The proper development of the fetus has obvious hormonal relationships, which are dependent upon fats.

Following birth, breast feeding helps protect the baby against allergies, asthma and intestinal problems through its high-quality fat content, particularly cholesterol. The baby is highly dependent upon the fat in the milk for survival, especially during the first few days. During this time, the fatty colostrum from breast milk is of vital nutritional importance.

### X-Ray Protection

Fats seem to help protect the body against the harmful effects of X-rays. This occurs through physical protection of the cell, and by controlling free-radical production, generated as a result of X-ray exposure. In addition to medical X-rays, we are constantly exposed to X-rays from the atmosphere. This cosmic radiation penetrates most objects, including airplanes. The average person gets more cosmic radiation exposure during an airline flight from New York to Los Angeles than from a lifetime of medical X-rays.

### Digestion

Because so many people digest their food poorly (a common result of stress), they do not always efficiently absorb the nutrients in foods. Your diet may be the best in the world but it's all for nothing if you can't properly digest and absorb the nutrients it contains. Bile from the gall bladder, triggered by fat in the diet, helps aid in the digestion and absorption of fats and fat-soluble vitamins.

Most of the fats in the diet are digested in the small intestine — a process that involves breaking the fat into smaller particles. The pancreas, liver, gall bladder and large intestine are also involved in the digestive process. Any of these organs not working properly could have an adverse impact on fat metabolism in general, but the two most important organs are the liver, which makes bile, and the pancreas, which make the enzyme lipase. If there is not enough fat in the diet, not enough bile will be secreted.

The secretion of bile into the small intestine makes dietary fat digestible. Certain lipase-containing foods such as avocados and extra-virgin olive oil can greatly aid digestion of fats.

Fat also helps regulate the rate of stomach emptying. Fats in a meal slow stomach emptying, allowing for better digestion of proteins. If you are always hungry it may be because your meal is too low in fat and your stomach is emptying too rapidly. Fats also slow the absorption of sugar from the small intestines, which keeps insulin from rising too high and too quickly. Additionally, fats protect the inner lining of the stomach and intestines from irritating substances in the diet, such as alcohol and spicy foods.

### Support and Protection

Fat offers physical support and protection to vital body parts, including the organs and glands. Fat acts as a natural, built-in shock absorber, cushioning the body and its various parts from the wear and tear of everyday life, and helps prevent organs from sinking due to the downward pull of gravity.

### Vitamin and Mineral Regulation

Most people know that vitamin D is produced by exposure of the skin to the sun. However, it is actually cholesterol in the skin that allows this reaction to occur. Sunlight chemically changes cholesterol in the skin through the process of irradiation to vitamin D-3. This newly formed vitamin D is then absorbed into the blood, allowing calcium and phosphorous to be properly absorbed from the intestinal tract. Without the vitamin D, calcium and phosphorous would not be well absorbed and deficiencies of both could occur. But without cholesterol, the entire process would not occur.

There's another important connection between calcium and fat. Calcium needs to be carried from the blood and taken into the bone or muscle cells. For this to happen certain prostaglandins, made from fat, are needed. If there is not enough fat to make adequate prostaglandins, too little calcium enters the bone. When that happens, the results can be stress fractures, osteoporosis and collapsed vertebrae. Without enough calcium in muscles, tightness, spasms or cramping can occur, since calcium is needed to relax muscles. Unused calcium may be stored, sometimes in the kidneys as stones, or in the muscles, tendons or joint spaces as calcium deposits, often called bone spurs.

Besides vitamin D, other vitamins, including A, E and K, rely on fat for proper absorption and utilization. These important vitamins are present primarily in fatty foods, and the body cannot make an adequate amount of these vitamins to ensure continued good health. In addition these vitamins require fat in the intestines in order to be absorbed. So a low-fat diet could be deficient in these vitamins to begin with and also could further restrict their absorption.

## Taste

My favorite function of fat is that it makes food delightfully palatable. Let's face it, people love foods with fat in them, but are so guilt-ridden about it, they just can't sit down at the dinner table and enjoy them. Fat does not have to be an unhealthy addition to your diet if properly balanced. It not only tastes good, but also makes you feel good — not just psychologically, but physiologically as well.

Fat also satisfies your physical hunger. People on low-fat diets often complain that they are always hungry. Of course they are. Without fat in their diet, they can't achieve a feeling of satiety. As a result, the brain just keeps sending the same message over and over: eat more, eat more. Because you never really feel satisfied, the temptation to overeat is irresistible. In fact, there's a good chance you can actually gain weight on a low-fat diet by overeating to try and get that "I'm not hungry anymore" feeling. Besides, low-fat meals can be extremely unappetizing, often leading to an unbalanced diet.

In addition, low-fat items typically have sugar added to make up for the reduced flavor.

## Brown and White Fat

The human body possesses two distinct types of body fat, referred to simply as brown and white. Both fat stores are active, living parts of the body, heavily influencing your metabolism. Most of your fat stores are white fat, making up 5 percent to as much as 50 percent of your weight. This fat serves mainly as stored energy.

Brown fat, however, makes up only about 1 percent of the total body fat in most individuals. But this type of fat helps regulate the fat-burning aspect of your metabolism, depending on how it is stimulated. It can make you gain weight and become sluggish in the winter like a hibernating animal. And, if your caloric intake is too low, brown fat can also slow the burning of white fat.

Brown fat is greatly controlled by temperature. If you get too hot during the day, or by overdressing when you exercise, you can decrease your brown-fat activity, leading to less burning of white fat. This is why wearing extra clothes or "sweat suits," during exercise, a common weight-loss myth, can be counterproductive. Even sitting in a hot tub, sauna or steam room regularly after exercise may offset some of the exercise benefits. It may increase sweating, which often results in some water-weight loss, but the sacrifice is actually less fat-burning.

In contrast, brown fat is stimulated by cold. Cooling your brown-fat areas can help stimulate more white-fat burning. Brown fat is found around the shoulders and underarms, between the ribs and at the nape of the neck. So end your shower with a minute or two of cool or cold water. And if you want to use the hot tub or sauna, take a cool or cold shower or tub bath afterwards.

Brown fat is also stimulated by omega-6 and omega-3 fats. The role of brown fat is just another of the many examples of healthy functions of fat in the body. But to make sure that the fat in your body is composed of healthy, balanced types of fats, you must be very careful with the types and amounts of fats you consume.

# 10 The Fat-Balancing Act

Now that we've cleared up some misconceptions about the importance of fat in your diet, we can focus specifically on how to balance different types of dietary fats to improve your health. The first thing to understand about fats is that, like carbohydrates, not all are created equal. The issue of different fats and their metabolism is quite complex; volumes have been written on the subject and many scientists have devoted their entire careers to this topic. There are many different types of fats with various chemical structures that come from many types of foods, and which do different things once inside the body. There are also many different methods of categorizing fats.

One categorization method is to adopt the standard that most people are familiar with, and which appears on most ingredient labels. This is to divide the types of fats into monounsaturated, polyunsaturated and saturated fats. This is actually helpful in some respects. As we shall see, the monounsaturated fats are associated with improved health and disease prevention, and should make up the bulk of fats in your diet. In addition, saturated fats and essential fatty acids from some polyunsaturated fats play an important role in balancing chemicals in your body that regulate inflammation, healing and other important bodily functions.

A few foods contain predominantly one type of fat or another, but most foods, even oils, contain a combination of all three. Many people are surprised to learn, for instance, that the fat in an average steak is about half monounsaturated and half saturated, with a small amount of polyunsaturated. Significant factors that may further determine the balance of fats in foods include the soil in which the food is grown and the feed on which the animal is raised.

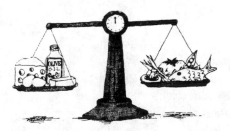

| Food | % Mono | % Poly | % Saturated |
|---|---|---|---|
| Olive oil | 77 | 9 | 14 |
| Canola oil | 62 | 32 | 6 |
| Peanut oil | 49 | 33 | 18 |
| Corn oil | 25 | 62 | 13 |
| Soybean oil | 24 | 61 | 15 |
| Safflower oil | 13 | 77 | 10 |
| Coconut | 6 | 2 | 92 |
| Egg yolks | 48.3 | 15.6 | 36.1 |
| Steak | 49.2 | 4.3 | 46.5 |
| Cheese | 30.1 | 3.1 | 66.8 |
| Butter | 30 | 4 | 66 |
| Almonds | 68.1 | 22.0 | 9.9 |
| Cashews | 61.6 | 17.7 | 20.7 |
| Peanuts | 50.6 | 31.6 | 17.7 |

The table above shows approximately how much of each type of fat is contained in some foods.

To simplify for our discussion, let's divide fats into two initial categories, and then further divide one of those categories. The first category of fats is the monounsaturated fats, which should make up about two-thirds of a healthy diet. The second category, which ideally comprises the other third of total fats in your diet, includes saturated fats and polyunsaturated fats. The polyunsaturated fats can be further divided into equal amounts of omega-6 and omega-3 fatty acids. You can simply picture your total fat consumption as a pie, such as in the accompanying chart.

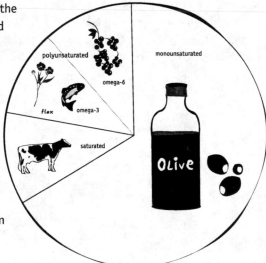

## Use Mostly Monounsaturates

As you can see from our chart, most of the fat in your diet should come from monounsaturated varieties. Extra-virgin olive oil, avocados and almonds are some good food sources of this fat. Monounsaturated fats are scientifically linked to many health benefits. The benefits of the Mediterranean diet, which include lower incidences of obesity and disease, are due in part to the fact that this style of eating is high in monounsaturated fat. The most important specific health benefit of monounsaturated oils is their association with cardiovascular health. Briefly, these fats are known to raise "good" HDL cholesterol and lower "bad" LDL cholesterol, as discussed in detail later in this book.

Another issue with fats is oxidation and the formation of oxygen free radicals due to exposure to air, light, heat and other factors. Excess free-radical production can lead to disease as is also discussed in a later section. Monounsaturated fats, however, are very stable and virtually immune to oxidation through cooking or through rancidity (due to exposure to air, light, etc.).

## The 'Champagne' of Oils

The best fat to use regularly is extra-virgin olive oil. In addition to its high monounsaturated fat content, it contains only about 9 percent polyunsaturated fat, making it one of the most stable oils.

As mentioned previously, monounsaturated oils have been associated with many health benefits. However, extra virgin olive oil is uniquely different from most other dietary oils, even other monounsaturated oils, in terms of its health benefits.

Extra-virgin olive oil is obtained from whole fruit by using the cold-press technique, which does not alter the natural antioxidants, phytonutrients or quality of the oil. The most potent phytonutrients are phenols, which give the oil its bitter-type taste, although more mature oils have a better, more fruity taste. Very high amounts of phenols are found in extra-virgin olive oil. Phytonutrients, including phenols, are virtually absent in almost all other oils, including olive oils that are not extra-virgin.

During the past few years, the actions of these phytonutrients have been extensively studied. Phenols can help reduce inflammation, and possess potent antioxidant properties. This antioxidant activity can prevent LDL cholesterol from oxidizing, which is what actually makes this "bad" cholesterol bad. These and other naturally occurring substances may also play a role in reducing blood pressure in those with hypertension.

Other studies show that extra-virgin olive oil can reduce the risk of some cancers, such as colon cancer, by influencing the metabolism of the intestines. Still other studies show that a diet high in monounsaturated fat may be preferable even to a low-fat diet in prevention of coronary heart disease since extra-virgin olive oil can raise HDL cholesterol.

When shopping for olive oil, survey the different brands as they vary greatly in taste. A visit to Balducci's in New York City's Greenwich Village will reveal many dozens of extra-virgin olive oils, all with different aromas, tastes and textures, not to mention prices. If you don't live near New York City, local Italian markets often carry several brands of imported extra-virgin olive oils.

Many people ask about the different grades of olive oil. Generally, you get what you pay for. Most imported olive oil is from Spain, Greece and Italy. It is graded by international standards, much like fine wine, for flavor, aroma and acidity. Extra-virgin is the tastiest and has less than 1 percent natural acid. Highly acidic oils (above 3.3 percent acidity) have an offensive taste and are neutralized by added chemical agents. In addition to extra-virgin, you may also see these grades of olive oil:

- **Virgin:** This grade is not readily available, and is often used to add flavor to lower grades. It contains between 1.0 and 3.3 percent acid, which adversely affects the taste. It is, however, still a good oil.

- **Pure:** The name can be misleading, as this is the lowest grade of olive oil available. The oil has been neutralized with chemicals to higher than 3.3 percent acidity, and has the least flavor. This grade of oil is not recommended for eating; if you have some on your shelf, it works well for squeaky doors.

- **Light or "lite":** These are oils marketed to people who think that fats are bad for them. It's just diluted pure olive oil, also something to be avoided.

By using mostly extra-virgin olive oil and other monounsaturated oils, as well as eating foods that are high in these health-promoting fats such as avocados and almonds, you will be well on your way to balancing your fat intake. For most people, a 2:1 ratio of monounsaturates to other fats will yield the right formula for greater health. To help you get on the road to more balanced fat intake I have included two recipes here — one for my Healthy Salad Dressing and another for Better Butter as follows. I have also included extra-virgin olive oil and almonds as ingredients in Phil's Bars™ and Alma bars™. But there's more to balancing your fats than just eating more monounsaturates. You must also balance the remaining fats in your diet — the polyunsaturated fats and the saturated fats. This is the subject of the next chapter.

---

**Phil's Healthy Salad Dressing**

Mix in a glass jar with tight-fitting lid:

- 8 ounces extra-virgin olive oil
- 2 cloves finely chopped garlic
- 2 ounces or more apple-cider vinegar
- 1 tablespoon fresh or dried parsley
- 2 teaspoons sea salt
- ½ teaspoon mustard

Option: Add 1 to 2 tablespoons plain yogurt, or sour cream.

Use other good-quality oils for variations in taste.

Shake well before serving. Refrigerate.

---

**Better Butter**

In a blender, mix two parts sweet (unsalted) butter and one part extra-virgin olive oil. Add sea salt to taste. Blend until smooth. Refrigerate and use as butter. After you acquire a taste for Better Butter, use half butter and half oil, or find the mix that suits your taste. Use a good-tasting extra-virgin olive oil for best results.

# 11 The ABCs of Polyunsaturated and Saturated Fats

The health benefits of monounsaturated fats are fairly simple to understand. However, the saturated and polyunsaturated fats that make up the other third of a properly balanced fat intake require a different level of understanding. These fats are responsible for the production of different types of important natural chemicals called eicosanoids. Eicosanoids include many different types of prostaglandins, leukotrienes and thromboxanes. But let's not get into that much detail here. For now just remember that balanced eicosanoids regulate certain bodily functions that are central to optimal human performance and disease prevention. Eicosanoid balance is one of the most important factors in preventing disease and living a long, healthy life. With this in mind, understanding the roles of polyunsaturated and saturated fats is as easy as ABC.

First let's define the three basic types of fat in this category as A fats, B fats and C fats. Each of these fats lead to the production of different eicosanoids, which serve specific purposes in the body.

A fats are found in highest concentration in vegetables and their oils, such as safflower, soy and corn. They sometimes are referred to by their chemical name, omega-6. These contain an essential fatty acid, linoleic acid (LA). Essential fatty acids are called "essential" because the body can't make them. You must get these from your diet or through supplementation — and without them you cannot be healthy. When consumed, LA is converted by the body to other fatty acids, including gamma-linolenic acid (GLA), a key substance for healthy metabolism. The end result is the series 1 eicosanoids, which are powerful substances for promoting and maintaining health. When A fats are required as a dietary supplement, food concentrates of black-currant-seed oil and borage oil are best because they already contain GLA.

The B fats that convert to series 2 eicosanoids include saturated fats and an essential fat, arachidonic acid (AA). B fats are found in dairy products such as butter and cream, and in meat, egg yolk and shellfish. The body can also make AA easily from A fats. AA, important especially for the developing fetus and for children, is categorized here with the saturated fats because it occurs mostly in foods containing higher amounts of saturated fats. However, AA is actually an omega-6 fat.

The C fats, chemically termed omega-3, are found mostly in ocean fish, beans, and the oils from flaxseed and walnuts. They contain alpha-linolenic acid (ALA), an essential fatty acid which is converted in the body to EPA (eicosapentaenoic acid) and finally to the series 3 eicosanoid group. Fish oils derived from cold-water ocean fish already contain EPA and are often used by people who require an omega-3 supplement. Flaxseed oil is also used as an omega-3 supplement, but does not contain EPA and therefore requires other nutritional factors to convert to EPA, as discussed later in this section.

Remember our pie chart from the previous chapter? We divided our total fat pie into two-thirds monounsaturated fats and one-third polyunsaturated and saturated fats. This smaller one-third portion must now be divided into three equal portions of omega-6 fats, saturated fats and omega-3 fats to properly balance the eicosanoids produced from these fats and to achieve greater health.

**A Question of Balance**
Any type of fat can be used for the production of energy. But the balance of A, B and C fats in the diet can have a significant impact on health and prevention of disease. You need approximately equal amounts of A, B and C fats in the course of a week, but not necessarily at each meal. By eating a balance of all three fats, you have an ideal ratio of polyunsaturated to saturated fats, 2:1, and you'll also be on your way to balancing all three series of eicosanoids. If you are a vegetarian, take in approximately an equal ratio of A and C fats; in this case, some of the A fats will convert to B fats.

Imbalances may occur due to consumption of too much of one type of fat and/or not enough of another. For example, if you eat too much meat and not enough vegetables, beans or fish, you may end up producing too many series 2 eicosanoids. As we'll see, an excess of series 2 eicosanoids is one of the most common fat imbalances. Certain foods, vitamins and drugs can also affect fat metabolism and eicosanoid production. In addition to unbalanced fat consumption, imbalances in eicosanoids can occur for other reasons:

- A lack of specific vitamins and minerals that are required for the conversion of A and C fats to their respective eicosanoids. These include vitamins B6, C, E, niacin, and the minerals magnesium, calcium and zinc.

- Certain dietary factors such as hydrogenated or partially hydrogenated fats, excess B fats, excess sugar and other carbohydrates, and low protein intakes can inhibit the conversion of A and C fats to eicosanoids.

- Lifestyle factors, such as stress and aging, which prevent or diminish formation of series 1 and 3 eicosanoids.

- Another important factor in eicosanoid balance is the real possibility that A fats will convert to series 2 instead of series 1 eicosanoids. This can occur when too many A fats are in the diet, when there's too much insulin production due to a diet too high in carbohydrates, and if you have too much physical, chemical or mental stress. In fact, most of series 2 eicosanoids come from A fats. Raw sesame oil, which contains the phytonutrient sesamin, can help prevent this from occurring.

| Factors that Help Series 1 & 3 Eicosanoid Production | Factors that Inhibit Series 1 & 3 Eicosanoid Production |
|---|---|
| Vitamins B6, C and niacin, low doses of vitamin E, magnesium, zinc and calcium, alcohol in moderation, black-currant-seed oil, fish oil | Hydrogenated fats, excess B fats, stress, aging, excess sugar and other carbohydrates, low-protein diet, cigarette smoke, fever |

## Eicosanoids and Inflammation

Perhaps the most important function of eicosanoids is their association with the body's inflammatory control mechanism. Inflammation is the body's way of responding to and repairing itself from daily wear and tear. Just going for a walk, working on the computer, washing the dishes, or any other repetitive motion, not to mention exercise, produces chemicals that cause inflammation as part of the body's complex recovery process.

The body continuously produces inflammatory chemicals. Once these inflammatory chemicals have done their work, anti-inflammatory chemicals are produced to stop the process. The reddish, swollen, hot area of a cut finger is an example of this normal inflammatory process.

The series 1 and series 3 eicosanoids produced from A and C fats have anti-inflammatory properties. Series 2 eicosanoids made from B fats have inflam-

| The Big Picture of ABC | | |
|---|---|---|
| **Type of Fat:** A (Omega-6) | B (Saturated) | C (Omega-3) |
| **Food source:** most vegetable oils | animal fats | fish, beans, flaxseed |
| **Contains:** linoleic acid | arachidonic acid | alpha-linolenic acid |
| **Converts to:** ⬇ | ⬇ | ⬇ |
| GLA ⟶ | | EPA |
| ⬇ | ⬇ | ⬇ |
| **Eicosanoid:** series 1 | series 2 | series 3 |
| **Response:** **anti-inflammatory** | **inflammatory** | **anti-inflammatory** |
| **Nutrition:** black-currant-seed and borage oils | — | EPA fish and flaxseed oils |

matory properties. In this example, it is clear how a balance of each is vital for good health.

Too much inflammatory chemicals, or not enough anti-inflammatory ones, can maintain inflammation, contributing to a variety of problems, including arthritis, colitis and chronic injury. As you will learn later in this book, over time this type of inflammation can lead to many dangerous diseases including cardiovascular disease, cancer, diabetes, Alzheimer's and others. In medicine, inflammatory conditions are treated with anti-inflammatory drugs, mainly because your body is not able to produce enough of its own anti-inflammatory chemicals. Otherwise you would not need the drugs.

### Other Functions of Eicosanoids

In addition to controlling inflammation, eicosanoids have many other important functions. Both series 1 and 3 chemicals decrease blood clotting and dilate blood vessels, which lowers blood pressure and increases circulation. In addition, these eicosanoids can reduce pain. Series 2 chemicals, however, do almost the opposite, constricting blood vessels and thereby increasing blood pressure and blood clotting. When out of balance, series 2 eicosanoids can trigger tumor growth, asthma and bone loss, increase pain sensation, and promote menstrual cramps.

However, do not allow yourself to think of B fats and their associated eicosanoids as bad. The B fats have, in recent years, been mistaken for "bad" fats. However, despite what the television commercials say, scientific evidence has not really implicated these as destructive to health when consumed as part of a balanced diet. In fact, a study published in the *American Journal of Clinical Nutrition* showed that people who consumed very high amounts of saturated fat, but who were active and did not consume excess calories, had a very low risk of cardiovascular disease. Unfortunately, modern social trends and the marketing of some food products form many misconceptions. For instance, margarine commercials are widely responsible for most people's false belief that margarine is more healthy than butter. And the media rarely reports the studies on the good aspects of fats and cholesterol.

The actions of B fats are essential. For example, without the constricting of blood vessels and the raising of blood pressure, blood circulation would be poor and not enough oxygen and other nutrients would be circulated throughout your body. Or, without blood clotting, you could bleed to death from a small cut. So don't think of "good" and "bad." Instead, think balance.

## Other Factors That Affect Eicosanoid Balance

Another important factor in eicosanoid balance is that B fats convert to series 2 eicosanoids very quickly and easily, while the transformation of A and C fats to series 1 and 3 eicosanoids requires numerous factors and has many potential inhibitors.

To produce series 1 and 3 eicosanoids from your dietary fats, certain nutrients are required. These include the vitamins B6, niacin and C, and low doses

## How Aspirin Works

In the conversion of A, B and C fats to eicosanoids, an important enzyme called cyclooxygenase is required. Aspirin, and all other non-steroidal anti-inflammatory drugs (NSAIDS), including Advil, Motrin, Naprosyn and Nuprin, temporarily block this enzyme, so much less of the inflammatory series 2 eicosanoids are formed. While this reduces the proinflammatory eicosanoids, these drugs also eliminate series 1 and 3 eicosanoids along with their beneficial properties. This may result in an improvement of symptoms, but it also turns off the important anti-inflammatory mechanism. In addition, the cause of the problem — often an eicosanoid imbalance — goes untreated. If aspirin makes you feel better, it may be due to the imbalance of your eicosanoids.

Ask yourself if you need to take drugs like aspirin or other NSAIDS to feel better. If they do make you feel better, you can be almost certain that your body is not making enough of its own anti-inflammatory chemicals. In other words, you have a possible imbalance of eicosanoids.

### Margarine: It's Not Nice to Fool Mother Nature

Since the 1950s, experts have questioned margarine's place in a healthy diet. The *New England Journal of Medicine* and other periodicals have more recently reported what many have thought for decades. Scientists have shown that eating hydrogenated fat, an ingredient found in most margarines, significantly increases the risk of heart disease by raising the LDL cholesterol, which is most responsible for fat deposits in the arteries, while lowering the "good" HDL cholesterol. The reason for this is the presence of trans fats contained in hydrogenated or partially hydrogenated fats. Trans fats also can disrupt eicosanoid balance and increase inflammation because they are handled by the body as saturated fats and converted to series 2 eicosanoids.

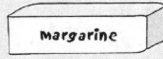

Manufacturers use the hydrogenation process to turn a liquid (e.g., soy oil) into a solid (margarine) product. But margarine is not the only product which contains hydrogenated fat. Read the labels of food packages: Many breads, crackers, chips, desserts and numerous other products contain hydrogenated or partially hydrogenated fats or oils. Avoiding them is easy — read labels and don't buy products that contain them. You can always find substitutes that don't contain these harmful substances.

---

of vitamin E in addition to the minerals magnesium, zinc and calcium. A small amount of alcohol, such as a glass of wine with meals, may also promote this activity.

There are many more factors that can inhibit the production of series 1 and 3 eicosanoids, with the most notable being consumption of trans (hydrogenated) fats, which are ingredients in many foods, including margarine. Other inhibitors include too many B fats, stress, high-carbohydrate diet, low-protein diet, cigarette smoking and fever. In addition, the normal aging process is accompanied by a slowing of series 1 and 3 eicosanoid production — all the more reason to be careful about your present lifestyle.

The process of eicosanoid inhibition is related to two enzymes (called delta-6-desaturase and elongase) which each convert A and C fats to series 1 and 3 eicosanoids. If there are not enough nutrients to help the enzymes convert either of these fats, eicosanoid production may be adversely affected. Taking concentrated sources of GLA and EPA may be beneficial, since they can bypass some of the potential inhibition. For example, black-currant-seed oil contains GLA, and fish oil contains EPA. Their conversion to eicosanoids is less likely to be inhibited.

**Do You Have an Essential-Fatty-Acid Imbalance?**
Certain signs, symptoms and lifestyle habits may offer powerful clues that your eicosanoids may be out of balance. The following survey can help you determine the likelihood that you have an imbalance in fats and eicosanoids.

☐ Aspirin or non-steroidal anti-inflammatory drugs improve my symptoms.

☑ I have chronic inflammation or "itis"-type conditions such as arthritis, colitis, tendinitis.

☐ I have a history or increased risk of heart disease, stroke, or high blood pressure.

☐ I often eat restaurant, take-out or fast food.

☐ I am intolerant to sweets and other carbohydrates.

☐ I follow a low-fat diet.

☐ I often feel depressed.

☐ I have a history of tumors or cancers.

☐ I sometimes suffer from reduced mental acuity.

☐ I have diabetes or family history of diabetes.

☐ I am over age 50.

☐ My blood tests show increased triglycerides or cholesterol.

☐ I have high insulin.

☐ I have spring allergies.

☐ I suffer from intestinal problems such as diarrhea, constipation, or ulcers.

If you checked one or more of these items there's a chance that you have an essential-fatty-acid imbalance. The more items you check off, the more likely you have a problem. Since omega-6 is prevalent in most diets, most people find they lack omega-3 fats. Diet adjustments including adding wild ocean fish, such as salmon, sardines, tuna, anchovies and mackerel, as well as almonds, walnuts, pecans and green vegetables, can be helpful in correcting an essential-fatty-acid imbalance. For those who cannot get enough omega-3 fats from the diet, supplements, such as Nature's Dose™ Infla-min Anti-Inflammatory Complex, are most effective. In addition, sesame-seed oil helps prevent omega-6 oils from being converted to arachidonic acid, thereby improving the balance of eicosanoids.

### How Fat Should Your Diet Be?

Equipped with the knowledge of how fats work in the body, especially their influence on the metabolism through eicosanoid function, you are in a position to improve your diet in accordance with your body's particular needs. How much fat should you have in a healthy diet? The amount of fat in a healthy diet depends on the individual.

You must first get over the idea that the less fat the better, or a diet that's 10 percent or 20 percent fat is ideal. Actually, a low-fat diet can be very unhealthy. For example, studies show that people following a very low-fat diet can increase their risks for heart disease. This is due to the fact that their intake of essential fatty-acids (the A and C fats) could be too low. There are many populations in which fat intake exceeds 40 percent, like the Eskimos and people living in the Mediterranean region, who on average are healthier than people in most populations who eat a lower-fat diet. In addition, the American Heart Association, the World Health Organization (WHO), the Surgeon General, the USDA and many other professional health organizations have recommended a diet that's 30 percent fat, not one that's 20 percent or even 10 percent.

I have found that most people are healthier with at least 30 percent fat in their diet. Some may need more — 35 or even 40 percent. But rather than follow these numbers, experiment and find what works best for you. In general, once you've found your optimal level of carbohydrates, and balanced your fats, the amount of protein you need to eat is fairly easy; this is the subject of the next chapter.

# 12 The Power of Protein

Once you've adjusted to the right amount of carbohydrates for your body, and added the proper balance of fats to your diet, proper protein intake is relatively easy to determine. For example, if you find that 45 percent of your diet is carbohydrate, and 30 percent is fat, the remaining 25 percent as protein would probably be the optimal amount for you. As convenient and oversimplified as that may sound, that's how it turns out for most people. Think of it as a puzzle; once you find the first two pieces, the third one falls neatly into place.

Growing children need higher amounts of protein for development. But once optimal body size is attained and growth stabilizes, there is still significant and continuous turnover of tissue protein. Even moderately active adults need protein to rebuild muscle tissue on a daily basis. In other words, throughout your life, your body continually makes new cells for your muscles, organs, glands and bones, all of which require protein as a main building block. Athletes or those who exercise require even higher protein intakes. In addition to growth and repair of muscles and other tissues, some protein is used for energy. The amount of energy contributed by protein may be as high as 15 percent for some athletes. Protein is also necessary for enzymes important to metabolism. Some of these important enzymes were discussed in the chapters on fats, specifically, the delta-6-desaturase and elongase enzymes necessary for the production of series 1 and 3 eicosanoids.

Protein is essential for maintaining neurotransmitters — the chemical messengers used by the nervous system to signal proper function throughout the body. Furthermore, oxygen, fats and vitamins are transported throughout the body with the help of proteins.

Protein is also necessary to make natural antibodies for the immune system. Those who lose muscle mass through reduced protein consumption have reduced immunity. And those who consume inadequate protein may not get enough of certain nutrients necessary for immune function. For example, the amino acid cysteine is contained in protein foods such as whey and can improve immune function. This amino acid is necessary for the body to make its most powerful antioxidant, glutathione.

## How Much Do We Really Need?
The debate about protein and its recommended daily allowance (RDA) has gone on for decades, with the RDA for protein being revised at least 10 times since 1943.

The most recent long-term studies indicate the USDA's recommended daily allowance for protein is simply not enough, especially for active adults and all those over 50.

Presently, many experts in this field feel the RDA of 0.8 grams of protein per kilogram of body weight is too low, with some suggesting three to four times that amount. Allow me to use grams of protein as an example of how much protein food is required in a day. This is only for comparison, and my amounts are all general. I don't want you weighing your food!

Using the USDA's minimum protein requirement for a 175-pound person, the daily protein requirement would be about 64 grams using the 0.8 g/kg formula. This amount of protein could easily be eaten from two eggs at breakfast, a turkey sandwich for lunch, and broiled salmon for dinner. And for a 145-pound person who requires about 53 grams: two eggs at breakfast, a small sirloin steak for lunch or dinner, and a handful of almonds for a snack. Here's another scenario providing that amount of protein for someone weighing 125 pounds, who would minimally require about 45 grams of protein: an egg at breakfast, tuna salad for lunch, and a small piece of cheese for a snack. Using the RDA values as the guideline — the minimum requirements — a significant number of people are protein-deficient. This is typical of what I saw when I was in private practice.

But what if you need more than the minimum requirement due to an active lifestyle? Or, what if many of the experts are right in saying we need two or even three times the RDA, or more? This brings into more precise focus how many people may not get enough protein. Consider the same meal plan for the three individuals in the preceding examples if the protein requirements are doubled. For our 175-pound person, if the total protein intake required became 128 grams, here are some examples of foods that would provide this: three eggs and ham at breakfast, a hefty turkey sandwich for lunch, and broiled salmon for dinner. For our 145-pound person, he or she might require about 106 grams: two eggs for breakfast, a chef's salad for lunch, and a sirloin steak for dinner. And for the person weighing 125 pounds, who would minimally require about 90 grams of protein: two eggs at breakfast, tuna salad for lunch, and pork roast for dinner.

This issue is somewhat distorted by the fact that using just body weight for protein requirements is not as accurate as using only the lean body mass — the total weight minus the body-fat weight. It's your lean body that needs the protein, not your stored fat. Using these measurements will often change the above requirements. See how complex this could get? I don't want you to get bogged down in such detailed analysis because it's not necessary; your body will tell you what to eat.

Some say that excess protein is dangerous. I agree; eating more protein than the body can utilize can be unhealthy. But if your body requires more than 100 grams a day, that's not excessive, it's what your body needs. Eating the amount of protein your body requires is not a high-protein diet, it's getting your requirements! But remember, as your protein intake increases, so does your need for water, which helps eliminate the by-products of protein through the kidneys. That's why some say that protein is a stress on the kidneys; it most certainly is if you are dehydrated. Many people are frightened away from eating enough protein by unfounded concerns, or by concerns that can be addressed simply by drinking enough water.

## Why So Much Confusion?

When determining protein needs, researchers measured the amount of protein taken in through food, then measured protein by-products to determine the amount lost. Many studies on protein requirements, especially research that established RDA levels, only measured the protein by-product nitrogen, excreted in the urine. They failed to consider the amount lost in sweat. This is clearly an important means for excreting the nitrogen from protein breakdown. Urea production alone may not accurately reflect all aspects of protein breakdown. This is one reason many earlier studies on protein requirements showed such low numbers. Other studies show improved physical function with diets high in protein compared to diets following RDA standards for protein. And enough experts have come to similar conclusions — that protein needs, including the RDA, for active people must be re-examined.

Whether you derive your protein foods from animal or vegetable sources, you still require a balance of protein, more specifically, of the different components called amino acids that make up protein.

## Amino Acids

Dietary protein is made up of building blocks called amino acids. In order to obtain these vital components, two important functions must take place. First, protein must be efficiently digested in the intestine, resulting in breakdown into amino acids. Second, these amino acids must be absorbed into the body. Once absorbed, the amino acids are used either as individual products, or recombined as proteins. For example, the amino acid tryptophan is used to make certain neurotransmitters in the brain. Or, recombining many amino acids provides for the manufacture of new muscle cells.

There are at least 20 amino acids necessary to human nutrition, all of which are indispensable for good health and fitness. While some of these amino acids can be made by the body, others must be taken in through the diet. Those the body can make are referred to as "non-essential," and those the body can't make are referred to as "essential." The following table lists both types.

| Essential Amino Acids | Non-Essential Amino Acids |
|---|---|
| Arginine | Alanine |
| Histidine | Asparagine |
| Isoleucine | Aspartate |
| Leucine | Cysteine |
| Lysine | Glutamate |
| Methionine | Glutamine |
| Phenylalanine | Glycine |
| Threonine | Proline |
| Tryptophan | Serine |
| Valine | Tyrosine |

It's important to note that arginine and histidine are sometimes called "semi-essential" since they are not made in adequate amounts in children. Also, some non-essential amino acids are made from essential ones. For example, tyrosine is made from phenylalanine, and cysteine from methionine (and serine). Most important is the fact that animal protein sources — meat, fish, cheese and eggs — contain all amino acids and are considered complete proteins. With the exception of soybean products like tofu which are complete proteins, vegetable foods individually contain only some of the amino acids. Combining the right non-animal foods can result in a complete amino-acid meal. But eating all the amino acids at one meal is not necessary. For those who don't eat animal products, obtaining all the amino acids is accomplished by combining enough variety, since no one vegetable-based food, except soy, contains all the amino acids. Any combination of whole grain and legume will provide a complete protein. For example, combining peanut butter and whole wheat, or rice and beans, provides a complete protein with all the amino acids.

The traditional amino-acid nomenclature is very misleading. Even though the non-essential amino acids can be manufactured by the body, the very real potential exists that some common metabolic problem, such as low magnesium or some other nutritional imbalance, may prevent the proper balance or amounts of these amino acids from being formed. This could result in amino-acid or protein problems. Essential amino acids merely need to be consumed in the diet, properly digested and absorbed.

In general, animal foods are the best sources of complete protein, containing essential and non-essential amino acids. Overall, the highest-rated protein food is eggs, followed by whey, beef and fish. In the following chapter we'll discuss some of these protein sources and the various health issues involved with their consumption.

# 13 Making Wise Protein Choices

Now that you know the importance of protein in the diet, you need to make good decisions regarding what protein foods you will eat. For most people getting enough protein should not be a problem. But there are many health choices to consider if you are going to eat eggs, meat and dairy foods.

For vegetarians, getting enough protein can be a challenge. Soy and certain combinations of legumes and grains can supply all essential amino acids. But if you can eat eggs and some dairy products, such as cheese, yogurt and whey, your task will be much easier.

For most of us, eating a variety of foods from real sources such as eggs, meat, fish, whey or soy is best. In this chapter I'll discuss various protein foods and recommendations for making healthy choices. You will often have the choice between higher- or lesser-quality items. For most people it will not always be possible to make the absolute healthiest choice. For instance it's not often that you'll find organic steak or eggs on the menu at a restaurant. Likewise, the chicken you buy from the grocery store may not always be free-range, and you may have to settle for a farm-raised salmon the next time you want grilled fish. Perhaps higher-quality protein items are not available or cost is an issue. The worst thing you can do is not eat protein foods at all. The best thing you can do is make the best decision most of the time. If your body is healthy, eating some less-than-perfect foods from time to time will have less negative effect. On the whole, however, it's best to decide to buy the highest-quality items available. Following is information and some suggestions to help you do that.

**The Incredible, Edible Egg**
Eggs are not just incredible, but what I would call the perfect food all wrapped up in one single cell. Yes, that's right, an egg is an individual cell. In this single cell, an egg contains the most complete and highest protein rating of any food, containing all essential amino acids. Two eggs contain more than 12 grams of protein, just over half in the white and the rest in the yolk. In addition, eggs also contain many essential nutrients, including significant amounts of vitamins A, D, E, B1, B2, B6, folic acid and especially vitamin B12. Eggs also contain important minerals including calcium, magnesium, potassium, zinc and iron. Choline and biotin, also important for energy production and stress management,

## Some Facts about Eggs

The taming of chickens and other fowl for egg production dates back to before 1500 B.C. in China. Today, eggs come in many sizes and shell colors, not just white and brown. Depending on the type of chicken which laid them, some eggs have tints of green, blue and red.

Eggs, of course, should always be stored in the refrigerator. Because of their porous shell, there is slight evaporation of moisture from the inner egg through the shell, which changes its flavor and freshness. If you are not using them quickly, store your eggs in a sealed container to prevent loss of moisture. Never store eggs next to highly flavored foods, such as onions and fish, because they will easily absorb these flavors. Always store eggs with the large side up, which suspends the yolk effectively within the egg white.

Chefs know that room-temperature eggs are easier to work with; when boiled, they don't crack, the whites are easier to whip, and the yolks "stand up" more when fried. If you're separating eggs, however, the colder ones are easier to work with. Speaking of boiled eggs, they should never really be boiled but kept just at a slight simmer until done. Furiously boiling them results in rubbery whites and less-tasty yolks. One way to prevent the shells from breaking during boiling is to use a pin. Prick the shell on the large end of the egg with a pin. This allows the air pocket, found in the large end of the egg, to escape during cooking. Otherwise, if the air can't escape, the pressure builds and it may crack the shell. The best way to cook soft- or hard-boiled eggs is to place them in cold water (½ inch above the eggs) and bring to a boil. Take off the heat immediately. For soft-cooked eggs, remove after 2-4 minutes, depending on your taste, and run under cold water. For hard-cooked eggs, cover and let sit for 15 minutes, then rinse in cold water and keep refrigerated until ready to use. (An egg that is less than two days old is very difficult to peel when hard boiled.)

Finally, before you buy eggs make sure they are relatively fresh by looking at the date. Or, you can shake them close to your ear; if you hear a sloshing sound, it means they've lost a lot of moisture over time and there's a big air space in them — avoid these. Eggs also contain a natural barrier — an invisible protective coating which keeps out bacteria. Never wash the eggs you're going to store because you will remove this natural protection.

are contained in large amounts in eggs. Most of these nutrients are found in the yolk of the egg.

The fat in egg yolks is also nearly a perfect balance, containing mostly monounsaturated fats, and about 36 percent saturated fat. And, egg yolks contain linoleic and linolenic acids — both essential fatty acids. Eggs have almost no carbohydrate (less than 1 gram), making them the perfect meal or snack for the millions who are carbohydrate intolerant. Ounce per ounce, eggs are also your best food buy with hardly any waste.

Most people love the taste of eggs, but many people are concerned about eating them because of cholesterol. In a later chapter you will learn that the cholesterol in eggs is not something to be feared, and how adding more eggs to your diet can actually decrease your risk of cardiovascular disease.

While eggs are one of nature's most perfect foods, they are only as healthy as the hens that lay them, since the nutritional make-up of eggs, especially the fat, is very dependent on what the chickens eat. For this reason you should avoid run-of-the-mill grocery-store eggs that have been produced in chicken factories. Unfortunately this includes most eggs on the market. The healthiest eggs are those that come from organic, free-range hens. This means that the chickens are raised on land that has been certified organic and the feed they are given is also organic. Free-range means that the hens are allowed to roam, and in doing so they generally will eat bugs and vegetable matter, thus the eggs yield a better fat profile, with more monounsaturated fat and more essential fatty acids.

If you can't find organic, free-range eggs, most groceries at least carry eggs that are either one or the other — organic or free-range. While organic and free-range eggs may cost a bit more than regular eggs, they remain a protein bargain. And if you can't find organic or free-range eggs? Regular old grocery-store eggs are still better than no eggs at all.

## Here's the Beef

It's no bull — if you want to be healthy, beef really is "what's for dinner." Consider that just 3 ounces of lean porterhouse is at least 70 percent water, yet contains 20 grams of protein, and just 6 grams of saturated fat, balanced by a healthy 7 grams of heart-friendly monounsaturated fat. In addition to being an excellent source of high-quality protein, beef is also rich in B vitamins, glutamine, calcium, magnesium, iron, zinc and other nutrients that are lacking in many diets.

Organic and natural beef have not been treated with antibiotics, growth-stimulating hormones or fed any type of animal-source protein common in most other animals. With the threat of bovine spongiform encephalophy, also known as "mad cow disease," it is especially important to buy beef that has not been given feeds that contain animal by-products. Organically raised beef cattle are fed only certified-organic feed and graze on organically certified land.

You can buy naturally raised meats in some grocery and health-food stores. Also check locally and on the Internet for farms and ranches that sell meat from animals that have been raised on natural feeds and without the use of growth hormones, antibiotics and other chemicals used by most stock-growers. Whether you live near a farm that sells natural or organic meat, or order from a ranch that does, you may wish to buy a side of beef so that you always have some on hand. The meat will keep well in a freezer until it's time to make another order.

When cooking beef, keep it on the rare side. Studies show that beef cooked medium, medium well, or well is associated with higher rates of stomach cancer. This is due to the production of carcinogens (herterocyclic amines) from naturally occurring creatinine during cooking. Heat-sensitive nutrients, such as the amino acid glutamine, are also significantly reduced in meat cooked beyond rare.

### The Poultry Flap

Recently the poultry industry decided to stop adding antibiotics to poultry feed. This action was based on evidence that bacteria in chicken and turkeys was becoming resistant to the drugs. The result is that when humans become infected with bacteria, antibiotics prescribed to them may be ineffective. This actions follows a measure in the 1950s banning the use of growth hormone in poultry.

While these actions are certainly steps in the right direction, there are still some concerns when it comes to eating chicken or turkey. The poultry industry has done such a good job telling you on paper how healthy chicken is over other meats, but few people really look at the way chickens are raised. Typically, more than any other animal, chickens are raised in very unhealthy environments. Today's chicken house is really a city, containing 100,000 birds or more, cooped up in tiny boxes or very crowded conditions.

Some chickens are treated with pesticides, and a government report says 90 percent have leukosis, a type of cancer. The USDA estimates that 40 percent of the chickens on the market are contaminated with salmonella. Worse is the fact that half of ground poultry contains salmonella but is allowed to pass USDA inspection. (Salmonella infection is recycled through the common practice of using waste chicken parts in the chicken feed.) I cite the chicken industry because it is by far the worst of the animal-food industries.

Most turkeys, like chickens, are raised in the unhealthy environments of poultry factories and are managed for quick growth rather than healthy table fare. In addition, some birds are injected after slaughter with unhealthy substances for flavor, color or to tenderize the meat.

All this does not mean that chicken and other poultry is not a good source of protein — you just need to find a good source. The best bird for the table is organically raised. This means that the animal has not been treated with or fed any chemicals or drugs, and has only been fed certified-organic feeds. This is the safest of all poultry. If you can't find organic poultry, free-range birds that have not been treated with pesticides, and which have been fed a diet that does not include animal by-products such as chicken parts, are your next best bet.

Many grocery stores and health-food supermarkets are beginning to carry organic, free-range and natural chickens and turkeys. In addition, you may be able to find birds such as these from a local farm.

## The Catch to Fish

Many people turn to fish as a healthy protein source. Fish are a good source of protein and some also contain significant quantities of essential fatty acids, especially omega-3 fats. However, just as with other protein foods, some fish are healthier choices over others. For instance if you are eating farm-raised salmon or other fish, your catch of the day may include antibiotics, pesticides, steroids, hormones and artificial pigments. In addition, pollution of waterways and oceans has increased the potential dangers of eating all fish and seafood.

Farm-raised salmon — which make up 95 percent of the salmon on the market and the bulk of fish purchased by consumers — are raised in aquatic pens, the undersea equivalent to cattle feedlots and chicken and hog factories. Since these fish are raised in confined, crowded and unsanitary conditions, the threat of disease and parasites is great. To combat disease and parasites, some fish farmers add antibiotics to salmon feed, and treat the salmon and their pens with pesticides. Some salmon are also treated with steroids to make the fish sterile, and growth hormones to speed them to market size and reduce production costs. In addition, since farm-raised salmon do not naturally eat crustaceans which make the flesh pink or orange, salmon growers often feed color additive to pigment the flesh.

If you choose to eat fish, it is best to buy wild-caught fish. This, however, is not perfectly safe either — one study found that more than 74 percent of wild fish caught near fish farms contained antibiotics from eating feed that drifted out of the fish-farm pens. In addition to feeds from fish farms, there are other concerns to eating wild fish. Contamination is possible due to infection from bacteria or viruses, heavy metals such as mercury, food additives such as sulfites and histamines, pesticides such as DDT, and other chemicals such as polychlorinated biphenyls (PCBs).

In general, avoid seafood that includes the so-called bottom feeders, those fish and other sea species that eat from the ocean's floor, where the potential for consuming toxic material is highest. This is especially true for those species that feed close to shore. Flounder, sole, catfish and crab are some examples of foods to avoid eating regularly. Oysters, clams, mussels and scallops are also sources of potential pollutants. Clams are perhaps the worst seafood to eat, especially when raw, since they normally filter out and concentrate viruses and bacteria, heavy metals and other chemical pollutants from the waters in which they live. If you enjoy eating seafood, here are some tips for doing so more safely and more nutritiously:

- Choose fish and crustaceans caught in waters farther away from polluted, industrial areas. Some examples are northern Maine lobster, Canadian salmon, sardines and herring.

- Look for cold-water fish like salmon, tuna, sardines and others which contain higher amounts of omega-3 fat and EPA.

- Eat smaller fish and crustaceans: trout, bass and shrimp rather than marlin and swordfish. Smaller and younger fish have not accumulated the toxins found in larger and older species.

- Avoid precooked fish, and prepared or processed seafood such as breaded fish or seafood, fish cakes, ground fish and imitation crabmeat.

- If you catch your own fish, ask local authorities about the limits of safety. Some regions recommend limiting how much of certain species you should eat in a year.

## Other Meaty Matters

In addition to beef, poultry and fish, other meats are also good sources of protein. Pork and lamb are popular meats, and recently more exotic meats such as buffalo have appeared in some groceries. When choosing these meats use the same guidelines as with beef and poultry — buy those that are raised naturally, or better yet, organically. A good deal of pork on the market is raised in large-scale hog operations, so, like chicken, it is advisable to look for better sources for this meat.

Wild game, including big-game animals such as deer as well as small game such as rabbits and game birds, is also another great source of protein. Wild-game meat is generally leaner but higher in essential fatty acids than domestic meats. While hunting your own meat is nearly ideal, there is a growing concern in some areas like the northeastern United States that the use of pesticides and other environmental chemicals has affected wild animals. But in general, wild game is much safer than store-bought meat.

One of the worst types of meat to consume is ground meat of any kind. Avoid all ground beef, poultry, pork or other meat, unless it has been freshly ground right before deep freezing or eating it. Ground meat is a haven for bacteria and can ferment in your intestine much worse than whole meat. If you like ground meat or have a recipe that requires it, it's best to buy a large piece of meat and then grind it up just before cooking — most butchers, even those in large groceries, will do this for you. Also beware of other meats that have already been cut, such as sliced meat, chopped meat and stew meat. Try to buy as large a piece of meat as possible and cut it yourself.

Processed meats can also be unhealthy choices. Most sausage, lunch

---

**Healthy Aspects of Animal Foods**

For most of their existence, humans have eaten significant amounts of animal foods — especially meat and fish, but also eggs. The human GI tract is well adapted for animal-food intake, having evolved on a high-meat, low-carbohydrate diet with varying amounts of vegetables, fruits and nuts. While the popular trend in recent decades has been toward the misconception that meat consumption is unhealthy, there are a variety of unique features of an animal-food diet that are vital for health and fitness. Here are some of them:

- Animal foods contain all essential amino acids.
- Vitamin B12 is an essential nutrient found only in animal foods.
- EPA, the most powerful fatty acid, and the one preferred by the human body, is almost exclusively found in animal foods.
- Iron deficiency is prevented by eating animal foods which contain this mineral in its most bioavailable form.
- Vitamin A is found only in animal products.
- Animal products are dense protein foods with little or no carbohydrate to interfere with digestion and absorption.
- People who consume less animal protein have greater rates of bone loss than those who eat larger amounts of animal protein.

meats and other processed meats are not only ground, but also may contain high amounts of sugar and chemicals that you don't want to eat. However, it is possible to find organic bacon and ham that have been cured with honey and with no harmful chemicals.

As odd as it sounds to most people, the most nutritious parts of the animal to eat are the organs and glands. In our society, the liver is the most common organ food, with stomach, brains, kidneys and others only rarely eaten. However, when a lion kills his prey, it's the organs and glands that are first devoured. The muscle, what we refer to as the "meat," is often left for the scavengers. Unfortunately, with our polluted environment, organ meats such as liver are becoming more dangerous since it's the liver's job to filter the blood and remove toxins from the body. If you enjoy liver and other organ and gland meats, be sure to find a good source, preferably organic.

### Say Cheese!

Cheese, cottage cheese and plain yogurt are dairy products that contain quality protein without many of the problems associated with milk. This is especially true if you can find products made from goat or sheep milk rather than cow milk. Goat and sheep milk are much more compatible for humans than cow milk.

Whichever type of milk they're made from, cultured products such as these are good sources of protein because the lactose, or "milk sugar," has been consumed by bacteria in the culturing process. These bacteria literally gobble up the sugar. To be sure that an item is fully cultured, check the "Nutrition Facts" on the label; the carbohydrate should be very low. This is also true of yogurt — many popular brands are not fully cultured. Of course you want to avoid the fruit-flavored varieties which are always full of sugar, with some containing more than ice cream.

If you use cheese, whole-milk cottage cheese or yogurt as protein sources it's important to remember that these are also high in B fat. So you must be careful to eat cheese in a way that maintains balance with your intake of A and C fats. In addition, since toxins often bind to fats, it's best to choose organic products. Avoid so-called "American" cheese, cheese spreads and other "process cheeses." These highly processed products, which outsell natural cheese, are usually several types of unripe cheeses, ground up with added chemical stabilizers, preservatives and emulsifiers.

Sheep and goat cheese and yogurt can be found in many supermarkets and health-food stores and are also available for order on the Internet.

## What's Up with Whey?

Remember Little Miss Muffet, eating her curds and whey? These are the two proteins found in milk. Whey protein is the thin liquid part of milk remaining after the casein (the curds) and fat are removed. Whey is the part of the milk containing most of the vitamins and minerals, including calcium. Whey is a complete protein. Its nutritional and therapeutic values are well documented, and this food is often referred to as a "nutraceutical."

Biothiols are a group of natural sulfur-containing substances that promote basic antioxidant activity in your cells, and are contained in high amounts in whey. In providing this vital raw material, whey is a key food for the immune system — one that can help prevent and treat many chronic conditions, from asthma and allergies to cancer and heart disease. It can also help improve muscle function.

The body uses the biothiols in whey as a raw material to produce a substance called glutathione. This substance is at the heart of regulating the body's antioxidant defense mechanism, and is even more important than vitamins C and E, and others in that group of popular antioxidants.

Those who are allergic to cow's milk can usually consume whey without problems. Small amounts of lactose are found in whey (much less than is found in liquid milk) but this is usually too little to cause intestinal problems, even in most people sensitive to lactose. In those who are truly lactose-intolerant (probably less than 5 percent of the population), this amount of lactose could be a problem.

Whey protein is contained in high amounts in certain cheeses, such as Italian ricotta; check the ingredient label on ricotta to make sure the main ingredient is whey. Whey also is a major ingredient in Phil's Bars™ and in Natural French Vanilla Phil's Shake™. Avoid highly processed whey products such as those which contain whey-protein isolate and caseinate.

## Myths and Facts about Soy

Soy is one vegetarian source of a complete protein. Whole green soybeans or edamame are excellent sources of protein and also fiber. Soy products such as tofu also contain quality protein. Soy protein such as that contained in Alma bars™ and Phil's Shakes™ is also a quality source.

When buying products that contain soy it is important to avoid those which have been highly processed. These include soy-protein isolates and caseinates and hydrolyzed soy, which often contain monosodium glutamate (MSG) as a by-product of processing. (This MSG by-product is not listed in the ingredients). Soy is acceptable as a food and food ingredient only if it reflects real soybean quantity and quality rather than a highly processed product. Examples of real soy foods include soybeans, tofu, and soy concentrates with the same amino-acid profile as whole soybeans.

Many people think soy is a wonder food. But like all foods, some people will benefit from soy while others may not. In fact, just as many people may be intolerant to soy as dairy. In addition, soy products fortified with concentrated isoflavones can pose serious dangers, including an increased risk of cancer, particularly for post-menopausal women, the very audience these products are marketed to by the big companies. They may also contribute to hormonal imbalance.

By choosing a variety of protein sources from the healthiest-possible eggs, beef, poultry, fish and other meats, as well as cultured dairy products, soy and whey, you will obtain a wide variety of other nutrients that also occur in these foods. For instance, eggs contain the important nutrient choline; beef contains L-glutamine; whey contains biothiols; and soy contains isoflavones. In addition, these foods also contain a variety of vitamins and minerals. But there's another food type that also is important in supplying vital nutrients. This vital food group, the vegetables, is perhaps the most important component to your diet and is discussed in the next chapter.

# 14 Vital Vegetables

So far we've looked in depth at the three macronutrients — carbohydrate, proteins and fats — as the basis of good nutrition. Now let's shift gears and take a look at a group of foods that really should have their own distinct classification — vegetables. Although vegetables contain varying amounts of all three classic macronutrients, they alone are as important to your health as all three combined and should make up the bulk of your food intake. Remember that at the beginning of this section I proposed a food pyramid with vegetables second only in importance to water. Vegetables contain antioxidant vitamins and minerals in doses as they were intended in nature. Perhaps even more important, vegetables contain phytonutrients, which many scientists believe may have an even more important role than vitamins in promoting health and preventing disease. Vegetables also contain protein and essential fatty acids, and are a key source of fiber and prebiotics, which are both essential for good health, as we will learn in the following chapter.

For this discussion, remember that fruits also contain many of the same nutrients as vegetables. Generally fruits are foods that contain a seed within, whereas vegetables have a separate seed. Though fruits also contain substantial micronutrients and phytonutrients, many are much higher in carbohydrate and so I usually consider these to be carbohydrate foods. However, there are some foods which are technically fruits that I categorize as vegetables — these include avocados, tomatoes, eggplant, peppers, squash and other fruits that are not sweet.

In our discussions of macronutrients in previous chapters we focused on amounts and ratios of macronutrients. When it comes to vegetables there's only one thing to remember: Eat as much of them as you can. While most people don't eat enough vegetables, there are very, very few who can eat too much of this good thing. I often recommend as a general guideline that people try to eat at least five servings of vegetables per day, including one raw, mixed salad. Seven or eight servings are even better. But what is a serving? Traditionally many have considered a serving to be a half cup. More recently, however, many dietary guidelines have recommended different approaches for measuring servings. For instance, a serving of lettuce might be a cup and a half; a serving of carrots might be one medium carrot; a serving of broccoli is one medium stalk, and a serving of asparagus is five spears. Using guidelines like these will help you to eat more vegetables than using the traditional half-cup serving.

## Vegetables: The Main Course

Many people think of vegetables as a tedious side dish. Actually you should consider vegetables your main dish. This may require adjusting the way you think about your meals. Think first what your main-course vegetable will be, and then make your other foods the side dishes — usually some sort of protein and an unrefined carbohydrate complete a balanced meal. In this way you can make vegetables the bulk of your diet.

Experiment in creating other types of meals around vegetables. For instance, a vegetable omelet with onions, red and yellow peppers and zucchini makes a meal out of eggs at breakfast. A vegetable-based organic-chicken soup with garlic, leeks, carrots, celery, and even green beans and yellow squash, is a bowl full of nutrition for lunch. Even Mom's meat loaf can be adjusted to include mainly vegetables — start with chopped onions, red or yellow bell peppers, zucchini, fresh parsley and garlic, and then add freshly chopped meat and season with sea salt and spices of your choice.

In choosing your vegetables don't overlook cooked greens. Some of the most neglected vegetables, such as kale, mustard greens, rapini, Swiss chard, collards, and the common spinach, are also some of the most nutritious. These bitter leafy vegetables are full of valuable phytonutrients, as well as a host of vitamins, including A and C, and minerals including calcium and magnesium. Once you get used to the idea of cooking greens, some meals just won't seem complete without them — truly, cooked greens can be served as a delicious bed for just about any protein food, from beef to fish. Greens can simply be steamed and served with a little butter or extra-virgin olive oil and sea salt. Or, add other vegetables to the mix, such as leeks, chopped white onions, mushrooms or red and yellow peppers. Cook your greens until they are slightly tender, but be careful not to overcook, lest you lose the vital nutrients. Just when they turn bright green is about right.

## Choose a Rainbow of Colors

In addition to eating enough vegetables it is important to eat a variety of these foods as well. The reason is that different vegetables contain varying amounts of specific nutrients. For instance a serving of leaf lettuce supplies 40 percent of the U.S. RDA of vitamin A, but only 6 percent of vitamin C. A serving of Brussels sprouts contains 110 percent of the RDA of vitamin C but only 10 percent of vitamin A. The same is true when it comes to minerals. Spinach, for instance, is relatively high in iron at 20 percent, but if it's calcium you're after you'll want to eat cabbage, broccoli, celery and green beans, each of which have 6 percent of the RDA per serving.

One of the easiest ways to ensure that you eat enough variety in vegetables is to use the "rainbow" technique. Choosing vegetables in a rainbow of colors will help ensure a variety of nutrients. For example, carrots and winter squash, which are orange, are high in beta carotene, which is converted by the body to vitamin A. Many green vegetables are high in vitamin C — a serving of broccoli, for example, provides a whopping 220 percent of the RDA! In addition to orange and green vegetables, consider purple eggplant, red radishes, white, green and red onions, white cauliflower, yellow summer squash, brown mushrooms and many others. Each of these colorful vegetables contains its own unique set of vitamins, minerals and phytonutrients.

**A Salad a Day**
In reaching your goal of five or more servings of vegetables per day, it's important to make sure some of this is in the form of a daily raw salad. Your salad can be a snack, a side dish or, with some added protein, it can be a meal in itself. Salad is a low-stress food, with little or no cooking involved and minimal cleanup. The base for a great salad, of course, is something green — fresh lettuce, spinach or even kale. Buy organic and buy often. The little bags of baby greens are fine so long as you eat them quickly. You can also buy whole heads of green- or red-leaf, Romaine, Bibb and endive lettuces. Then, for a few days of really quick salads, clean a whole head of lettuce, dry the leaves well (spinning works great), and refrigerate them in an airtight container with a piece of paper towel. Your lettuce will be ready to go when you need it.

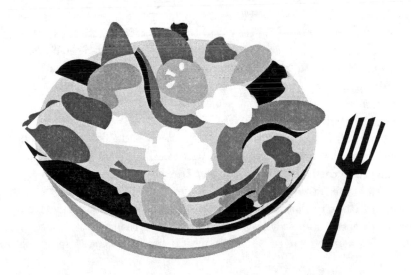

You may have heard the joke about the Honeymoon Salad — "Lettuce alone!" That's okay for newlyweds, but don't get caught regularly with just greens. Add a variety of raw vegetables such as carrots, chopped red and yellow peppers, purple cabbage, tomatoes and avocados. Steamed and chilled green beans and asparagus also liven up a salad. Chopped walnuts, slivered almonds, piñon nuts, gourmet olives, capers and artichoke hearts make a salad even more exotic.

To make your salad into a true meal, add some protein. Grilled tuna, wild shrimp, sliced beefsteak, hard-boiled eggs or shredded goat cheese are some options. Of course, a great salad requires a delicious dressing. Phil's Healthy Salad Dressing as described in chapter 10 is great, but simple extra-virgin olive oil and vinegar is fine too. Make your own dressing and avoid the additives that come out of a bottle.

**The Bitter Truth**

It's now clear that naturally occurring substances known as phytonutrients, or phytochemicals, found in vegetables and fruits, may be more important to good nutrition than vitamins, and can help prevent and treat cancer and other diseases. Their actions halt the production of cancer-causing agents in the body, blocking activation of these chemicals, or suppressing the spread of cancer cells that already exist. So the first step is eating your vegetables and fruits. The vegetables and fruits researchers think are most capable of preventing cancer and other diseases, including heart disease, are green leafy vegetables, broccoli, Brussels sprouts, cabbage, onions, citrus fruit (not just the juice), grapes, red wine, green tea and others. The more bitter, the better.

How many times have you heard that if something tastes good then it must not be good for you, or vice-versa? While this is a gross generalization, it's a fact that many people avoid eating bitter-tasting vegetables and fruits, which are particularly high in the natural disease-preventing phytonutrients that cause their bitterness. In general, the more bitter the taste, the more rich the food is in these phytonutrients.

For plants, these bitter-tasting substances — the healthy phytonutrients — serve as natural insect repellents and pesticides. Some are even toxic to rats, including some compounds in cabbage and Brussels sprouts. Generally, higher amounts of bitter-tasting phytonutrients are found in sprouts and seedlings than in mature plants. This provides young plants with a type of natural protection from being eaten at an early stage of life, before the chance of reproduction. While these nutrients can be harmful to insects and small animals, much the same way concentrated soy isoflavones found in many products can be harmful to humans, the therapeutic value of phytonutrients found in whole foods is unrivaled by nutritional supplements. And a human would have to consume pounds and pounds of vegetables daily to ingest toxic amounts of phytonutrients.

Despite the therapeutic and nutritive value of phytonutrients, the food industry is solving the so-called "problem" of bitterness in fruits and vegetables by removing these healthful chemicals through genetic engineering and selective breeding. Unfortunately, our culture has associated bitterness with bad taste instead of health promotion. Now many agricultural scientists, who consider some phytonutrients "defects" of nature, are changing our food supply for us — they are literally removing the healthy components from certain foods in order to sell more food products. And they are succeeding. Canola oil, for example, contains significant reductions of phytonutrients due to selective breeding. And transgenic citrus is now a reality — it's sweeter, but it's also free of limonene, the bitter substance that can help prevent and treat skin cancer.

Cancer researchers propose that a heightened sense of bitterness might be a healthy trait, allowing people to select foods with the highest phytonutrient content. This view contrasts with the food industry's practice of measuring the content of these bitter phytonutrients merely as a way of developing new non-bitter, phytonutrient-deficient strains. So while some nutrition scientists propose enhancing phytonutrients in foods for better health, the standard industry practice has been to remove them for better taste. Indeed, the lower amount of bitter compounds in the modern diet reflects the "achievement" of the food industry. The irony is that as agricultural scientists remove more phytonutrients from plants, farmers have to use even more chemical pesticides to protect their crops; thus consumers are left with the double-whammy of vegetables and fruits with less nutrition and more harmful pesticides.

In addition to bitterness, an astringent taste is also associated with healthy phytonutrients. These tastes can actually be quite attractive. Consider a fine aged Bordeaux or a high-quality green tea. Unfortunately, these are exceptions, and sweetness is a dominant taste preference, or perhaps "addiction" is a better word.

You can get more phytonutrients into your diet by eating foods that have a natural bitter or astringent taste. Zucchini and other squashes, pumpkins, cucumbers, melon, citrus, and many other vegetables and fruits, along with almonds and many types of beans, contain natural phytonutrients, as do red wine, green tea and cocoa.

### Is "Certified Organic" Worth the Price?

Today consumers are more and more likely to see certified-organic produce in grocery stores, and are faced with the decision over whether it's worth the extra price to buy these higher-quality items (although sometimes organic produce is about the same price as conventional). My feeling is that it is definitely worth the higher price to buy organic whenever possible, for many reasons. Organic produce usually tastes better, has not been genetically altered, and contains much smaller amounts of chemical fertilizers, or none at all. Moreover, many studies indicate that organic produce is more nutritious, containing more vitamins, minerals and phytonutrients.

For years, nutritionists insisted that today's conventionally grown foods were as high in vitamins and minerals as the meals of our grandparents. There is now sufficient evidence indicating this is not necessarily the case. Reductions in food quality have taken place since the mid-1940s, when the use of chemical fertilizers and pesticides rapidly became the norm in U.S. farming. A study in the *British Food Journal* compared the 1930s nutrient content of 20 fruits and vegetables with foods grown in the 1980s. Significant reductions were found in the levels of calcium, copper, and magnesium in vegetables; and magnesium, iron, copper and potassium in fruit. Similar trends can be found in foods produced in the United States, with reductions in some nutrients of as much as 32 percent.

While it's not widely believed that certified-organic foods are more nutritious, a recent study by Dr. Virginia Worthington, while at John Hopkins University, showed that vitamin C, iron, magnesium and phosphorus were higher in organically grown foods compared to non-organically grown foods. The levels of some nutrients were higher by nearly 30 percent. My own research has shown that some organically grown vegetables had significantly higher levels — 10 times or more — of certain nutrients such as folic acid, compared to the same vegetables tested and listed in the USDA database. The various studies analyzed many vegetables, including carrots, cabbage, lettuce, kale, tomato and spinach, with apples and pears included in the fruits that were studied. The increased nutrients found in certified-organic vegetables and fruits are most likely due to better care of the soil by organic farming methods, including composting, crop rotation and cover crops. Not all nutrients have been tested in these studies.

Just how these differences could affect health may be difficult to answer, but clearly we may be getting less nutrition from our non-organic food supply. Dr. Worthington states, "For vitamin C, in particular, five servings of the organic vegetables met the recommended daily intake of 75 mg for women and 90 mg for men whereas the same vegetables produced conventionally failed to do so."

Almost all foods are farmed with chemical fertilizers and pesticides, with the exception of certified-organic foods. Certified-organic foods contain significantly less nitrates and heavy metals, both of which can be very harmful, especially to children. Heavy metals enter the plants through certain chemical fertilizers — some of these fertilizers are even derived from industrial waste.

As discussed previously, phytonutrients, which are so important in a natural diet, are also genetically engineered out of some common foods to make them less bitter. Organically grown foods don't contain genetically engineered foods or genetically modified organisms, making them a better choice.

Then there's another factor to consider when choosing organic produce. Today much produce is imported. The countries of origin may not have as stringent restrictions regarding the use of fertilizers and especially pesticides as we have in this country. In fact, some countries still allow the use of pesticides that were banned decades ago in the United States. Choosing organic produce eliminates this potential problem.

While there are plenty of good reasons to choose organic, it may not always be possible. Just as when choosing other foods, try to eat the healthiest-possible option every time, but don't be overly concerned if you happen to eat non-organic vegetables from time to time due to availability or price considerations. Eating non-organic produce is still, on the whole, better than eating no produce at all. But pay attention to certain vegetables. Celery, for instance, has a tendency to retain chemical residues more than other vegetables. And some vegetables, such as leafy greens, are often more heavily sprayed than others.

If you really want the highest-quality produce, the best option is to grow your own. If you have any yard space at all, a small vegetable plot, properly tended, can yield enough vegetables in season for your entire family. By growing your own vegetables you can ensure their quality, reduce the price of your produce habit and revel in the enjoyment of producing your own food, not to mention the extra exercise you get from working in your garden.

It's clear that Mom was right when she told you to eat your vegetables. This important group of foods truly deserves its own classification. Eat as much of as many types as you can, both cooked and raw, and choose organic whenever possible. Making these healthy vegetable choices is just another journey on the road to better health and fitness, and also will help ensure that you get enough of another important food group, fiber and prebiotics, which are the topics of our next chapter.

# 15 The Full Spectrum of Fiber

Vegetables, fruits and other plant materials contain certain types of food particles that are not digestible or absorbable, but have powerful health-promoting effects. These include fiber, which improves function of the colon, a part of the large intestine, by promoting bulk. In addition, prebiotics, which are similar to fiber, promote the growth of healthy bacteria in the colon. Fiber and prebiotics have a symbiotic relationship that not only promotes healthy colon activity but also is important to overall body function.

Dietary fiber and prebiotics are found in vegetables, fruits and grains and are the elements that give structure to the cell walls of these plant foods. Various types of fibers have different names, depending on the part of the plant and type of plant from which they are derived. It's important to eat a variety of fiber-rich foods in order to obtain the full spectrum of these fibers. They include pectin, cellulose, beta-glucans, mucilages and a variety of gums including guar, arabic and locust bean.

Pectin is the substance partly responsible for the ripening of fruit. It is especially high in apples, grapes, citrus and most berries and is used as a gelling agent in foods such as jam. Applesauce is a high-pectin food that works as a remedy for diarrhea by adding bulk to the intestinal contents. Cellulose, such as found in wheat bran, is a component of cell walls of most plants. Beta-glucans from oats have become popular because of their positive association with reducing the risk of cardiovascular disease. Mucilages, such as psyllium and seaweed, are very functional fibers that are rich in minerals. Natural gums, as extracted from certain plants, have been used for thousands of years as thickening agents and emulsifiers, and they also prevent sugar from crystallizing in food products.

It's not so important to remember all the different names of these natural fibers. But it is important to remember to eat a variety of vegetables and fruits, which will provide you with the full spectrum of fiber important not only for your intestines but for your entire system. When, and if, you eat too much of one particular type of fiber, and consume it apart from those in natural foods, you risk creating an imbalance. It's analogous to the ABCs of fat — balance is the key. Try to get all the fiber you need by eating a variety of vegetables and fruits. At least one, preferably two or even three, semi-solid bowel movements (that float rather than sink) per day is a general indication that you're eating enough fiber.

If you still need more fiber after eating as much fiber-rich food as possible, you can supplement your diet with additional concentrated sources. Different people respond differently to specific types of fiber, but generally psyllium performs very well in most people. It is important to re-emphasize that eating a variety of fibers through fruits and vegetables will ensure you receive what your body requires.

If you need help remembering to eat a variety of fiber, there's the "45 Rule." Your intestines can store as much as 45 pounds of waste if it's not eliminated daily. Up to 45 percent of the weight of your stool may be made of bacteria — the good type that grows in your colon when you eat good food that includes the right fibers.

## Physical Aspects of Fiber in the Intestine

Fiber, by definition, is not absorbable. This has certain specific and important implications for the intestines. First, fiber acts as a vehicle, helping to transport food through the intestines at a healthy rate. The more-rapid transit time that results from fiber in the diet also limits the amount of time cancer-causing chemicals are in contact with the intestine's cells. After the body absorbs whatever nutrients it can get from the non-fiber portion of the meal, that food (now referred to as waste) is eliminated via the large intestine with great assistance from fiber. Fiber also affects the viscosity of the food, beginning in the stomach, and controls the rate of digestion. Too little fiber results in a too-rapid digestion in the upper intestine.

Fiber also is capable of holding water in the intestine, which has an important function of diluting potential toxins, including carcinogens, and preventing constipation. These toxins may also attach to the fiber and be removed from the body.

In the large intestine, fiber creates and provides the proper environment for the growth of "friendly" bacteria, which have a very important function. These micro-organisms ferment some of the fiber substances, improving the health of the intestine and other areas of metabolism. Intestinal bacteria also produce important fatty acids. These fats regulate the acid-alkaline balance in the large intestine and in turn control the bacteria themselves. Some fatty acids serve as an important energy source for the cells in the lower intestine. One specific fatty acid, butyric, may also play a protective role against cancer by maintaining a low colon pH and directly inhibiting tumor formation.

The process of fermentation also results in intestinal gas (mostly hydrogen and methane). If there's too much gas, causing discomfort or pain, it's a sign that there's a problem. Some of this gas is actually absorbed via the large intestine into the body, and is released through the lungs. Those individuals with bad breath usually have too much fermentation or gas from unfriendly bacteria. In any of these instances, stress, the wrong foods (such as too much carbohydrate) or too little fiber, among other problems, can be the cause. Antibiotic use, which kills the friendly micro-organisms in the intestine, can also be a cause. This destruction of the normal bacteria results in a "recolonization" of the large intestine with unfriendly bacteria. Yogurt, which contains friendly bacteria, can be helpful in these situations, as can L-glutamine supplements that contain lactobacillus and other healthy organisms. Furthermore, eating foods that contain prebiotics helps promote the growth of healthy bacteria in the colon, as discussed later in this chapter.

The effect of fiber on bile may also be related to the prevention of colon and rectal cancer. Excess amounts of bile in the colon may cause normal cells to convert to cancerous ones. By eating enough fiber and enough variety of fiber, the concentration of bile in the colon remains lower.

## Fiber and Absorption of Nutrients

Another important function of fiber is how it affects the absorption of nutrients from your diet. For example, fiber in your meal can reduce glucose absorption, and lower the glycemic index of that meal. Remember that the glycemic index is a measure of the blood-sugar response to certain foods or meals. Fiber-rich foods generally have a lower glycemic index and when consumed result in less insulin production. This makes fiber especially important for anyone with carbohydrate intolerance. Pectins, mucilages, and especially gums, seem to do this very well.

Absorption of minerals is also influenced by fiber, but in a negative way. Phytic acid, a natural substance present in the fibers of grains and in smaller amounts in fruits, can inhibit the absorption of calcium, iron, zinc and copper, and possibly other nutrients. For those who may have problems getting enough of these minerals, limiting grains and fruits can be helpful.

In addition to their relationship to mineral absorption, some fibers may have an adverse effect on digestive enzymes. Wheat bran, for example, can inhibit the production of pancreatic enzymes responsible for digesting carbohydrates, proteins and fats. The fiber in legumes may inhibit the enzyme amylase, which is important for carbohydrate digestion. Other studies show that the fiber in many cereals contains pancreatic inhibitors that can diminish protein digestion. In addition, the fiber in unprocessed soybeans can induce an allergy-type reaction in some people, accounting for the intestinal discomfort some may have with unprocessed soy. Normal intakes of most fiber types should not be a concern. But overconsuming — eating more than your body needs — can cause problems.

### Energy from Fiber

Since fiber is not absorbed, it does not directly count as an energy source. For this reason, if you eat a slice of whole-grain bread that contains 15 grams of carbohydrate, you really can't count it as 15 grams of usable energy, since some of that carbohydrate is fiber. If that slice of bread contains four grams of fiber, subtract four grams from the 15 grams of total carbohydrate, giving a total of 11 grams of usable carbohydrate.

While the fiber grams are not directly counted as energy calories, the body does indirectly obtain energy from fiber through fermentation by bacteria in the large intestine. As mentioned previously, fiber provides the environment for this bacterial activity. The bacteria produce short-chain fatty acids, typically butyric, acetic and propionic, which are absorbed and used by the body as fuel. Some fibers, such as pectin, are more capable of producing energy than others, such as fiber from grains. Approximately two calories of energy can be produced per gram of fiber. This is compared to four calories for other dietary carbohydrates, four for protein and nine for dietary fats.

### Prebiotics — the Other 'Fiber'

Most of us have heard about the many benefits of dietary fiber, but certain fiber-like foods called prebiotics can even more dramatically improve the function and health of the colon. Prebiotics include one group of natural non-digestible carbohydrates called fructans. Fructan-rich foods should be eaten daily, if possible. Fructans are contained in small amounts in most plant foods, but high levels are found in asparagus, onions, leeks, garlic, chicory and bananas. Dandelion greens are one of the highest sources of fructans, as are Jerusalem artichokes, or products made from them. Barley, rye and wheat are also good sources, although wheat comes with its own set of other drawbacks as discussed earlier.

Fructans act similarly to fiber, but do not actually create bulk themselves; instead they promote bulk by encouraging the growth of healthy bacteria in the colon — as much as popular probiotics such as acidophilus cultures in supplements and yogurt. In many people, prebiotics can actually help healthy colonic bacteria replace unhealthy bacteria that commonly cause disease.

While improved colon health can help prevent constipation, diarrhea and other functional problems, it can also help prevent intestinal diseases including cancer, and serious inflammatory conditions such as ulcerative colitis and Crohn's disease. Other bodywide benefits may include prevention of heart disease, other cancers and even osteoporosis. In addition, fructans help the colon produce certain nutrients, including biotin, vitamin K and some of the B vitamins. As opposed to some fibers, such as wheat fiber, which can prevent calcium, iron and other minerals from being absorbed, fructans can actually improve mineral absorption. This is the reason for a positive relationship between fructan intake and prevention of osteoporosis.

Since cooking can reduce the availability of prebiotic foods by 25 to 30 percent, try to eat enough raw vegetables, such as onions and garlic (which also have other health-promoting properties when eaten raw). Loss of fructans occurs in cooking water, so when cooking these foods be sure to consume the water too.

Fructan supplements have appeared on the market over the last few years, as both inulin and oligosaccharides. The natural version of inulin is extracted from chicory root using only hot water, filtration and drying. Unfortunately, most versions are highly processed, and have been synthesized from sugar. Synthesized fructans are also used in the manufacture of fake food ingredients — both for artificial fats and low-carbohydrate foods. For most people, obtaining sufficient fructans can be accomplished by eating more foods containing them.

### How Much Do You Need?

So how much fiber and prebiotics should you eat? By now you should know the answer to this question — it depends on your individual needs. On average, between 15 and 25 grams of fiber per day is the absolute minimum most people require. This works out to be about 10 grams per 1,000 calories. Many people need more fiber than this, and some people may need twice this much, or even more, to have optimal health.

Prebiotics should not be counted as part of the fiber requirement — instead, they should be consumed in addition to fiber. The symbiotic relationship of prebiotics and fiber mean that consuming proper amounts of these substances will improve the functionality of both. While there are no specific recommendations for the amount of prebiotics you should consume, Americans eat on average only about 1 to 3 grams of fructans daily, while our healthier European friends consume three times that amount. This does not necessarily mean that more is better, but most people will benefit by eating more food fructans.

If you don't get enough fiber naturally from foods in your daily diet, you may need a dietary supplement. The best way to do this is to make your own mix of fibers. This may require some experimentation, but it will be worth the effort. For example, you may try a mixture of psyllium and oat bran, mixed with applesauce (a good source of pectin). A quick analysis of your diet should give you an idea of how much fiber you're getting, and how much more you'll need. For many people who are carbohydrate intolerant, a supplement of fiber may be necessary.

Aside from eating enough fiber, it's also important to spread your fiber consumption out over the course of the day. In other words, you don't want to consume the bulk of your fiber by itself in one meal or snack. Eating meals and snacks that include a variety of fruits, vegetables and other fiber- and prebiotic-rich foods throughout the day ensures these importance substances will mix with your other foods to maximize the healthy benefits.

# 16 Water, Water Everywhere

The three macronutrients — carbohydrate, protein and fat — are often the key focus in discussions on nutrition. In this book, we've expanded on those to discuss vegetables and fiber as other very important dietary components. But there's another nutritional component that's even more important than all of these together. This nutrient is water. Pure, clean water is the most essential of all nutrients. You can live for weeks without consuming food. But go more than a couple days without water and your very survival will be at risk. Proper intake of water is so vital to optimal function that a deficiency of less than 1 percent can begin producing signs and symptoms of dysfunction. Slightly more dehydration can produce significant health problems. The key to maintaining proper hydration is to drink plenty of water throughout the day.

Water is the key ingredient in maintaining chemical balance in your body. This includes transporting nutrients to the cells, maintaining the function of blood, and eliminating wastes from the lungs, skin and colon. Water also plays a major role in hormone regulation and balancing acid-base levels. More importantly, water is like your car's radiator, cooling the reactions that create heat in your body. For example, muscle contraction, digestion and the processing of nutrients produce large amounts of heat, which must be cooled by water. If this regulation did not occur effectively, your temperature would rise to a level that would destroy your enzymes and other protein-based substances, and you would die. The water literally absorbs the excess heat and carries it to the skin, where it is dissipated through evaporation and other means.

About 60 percent of the body is made up of water, with different areas accounting for various percentages. For example, about 80 percent of your blood, heart, lungs and kidneys is water; your muscles, brain, intestines and spleen are about 75 percent. Even areas like your bones, which are 22 percent water, and fat stores, 10 percent water, require a specific level which, if not maintained, results in poor function.

One of the biggest problems of dehydration is that it decreases blood volume. Maintaining blood volume is important because so many vital functions are associated with it:

- Transport of oxygen-carrying red blood cells to the muscles.

- Transport of nutrients, including glucose, fats and amino acids.

- Removal of carbon dioxide and other waste products.

- Transport of hormones that regulate muscular activity.

- Neutralization of lactic acid to maintain proper pH.

- Maintenance of efficient cardiovascular function.

Most of the body's water is contained inside the cells of muscles, nerves, organs and even the bones. This water helps regulate the intracellular environment. Water also functions in between the cells by helping to carry nutrients and hormones into the cells. One of the most significant functions of water is to regulate the balance of potassium (on the inside of the cell) and sodium (outside the cell). This balance is most important in nerve and muscle cells, producing nervous-system function and muscle contraction.

**Preventing Dehydration**
Thirst is how most people remember to drink water. But this is a problem, since the brain's thirst center does not send a message until you are almost 2 percent dehydrated. By then, you already have problems associated with dehydration. The kidneys, however, respond to dehydration much sooner than the brain tells you you're thirsty, another good example of your body giving you signals. In this case, if your urine output is diminished, you're beginning to dehydrate. What is meant by diminished? If you're not urinating at least six to eight times each day, you may be dehydrated. In addition, the color of your urine also tells how well you're hydrated. Your urine should be clear. If your urine is yellow, it probably means you need more water.

Water input must balance water loss, which occurs from several areas of the body. Most water is lost through the kidneys. This water is used to help eliminate waste products from the body. But during vigorous activity, such as exercise, the body attempts to conserve water, and loss through the kidneys is very limited. Evaporation from the skin, important for controlling body temperature, is also a major source of water loss. Even under cool, resting conditions, about 30 percent of water loss occurs here. But sweating, from exercise or normal daily activity, increases this amount dramatically — during exercise, it's about 300 times the amount lost during rest! Water loss in exhaled air is also significant. The air going in and out of your lungs needs to be humidified. And a small but significant water loss (about 5 percent) occurs through the intestine.

The amount of water loss is determined in part by air temperature (the higher the temperature the more water loss), humidity (drier climates result in more water loss), and body size (the larger the person the more water loss). If you're dehydrated, just drinking a glass of water won't solve the problem. Complete water replacement may take 24 to 48 hours no matter how much you drink at one time. Unfortunately, the human body does not function like that of many other animals. By drinking a large volume of water, dehydrated animals can consume 10 percent of their total body weight in a few minutes, and rehydrate. Humans need to drink water in smaller amounts much more frequently to correct dehydration and maintain proper hydration.

What should you do to prevent dehydration and maintain proper hydration? Here are some general everyday guidelines:

- Don't wait until you're thirsty to drink water. Drink water every day, throughout the day.

- Drink smaller amounts every couple hours rather than two or three large doses a day.

- Have a water bottle near you at all times, and get into the habit of drinking water. Especially keep water near your immediate area during work hours or where you spend much of your time (at your desk, by the phone, in your car).

- Avoid carbonated water as your main source; the carbonation may cause intestinal distress.

- Get used to drinking water before, during and immediately after exercise.

- Learn to drink water without swallowing air.

- Remember that the average person may need about three quarts of water each day.

- Avoid chlorinated and fluoridated water.

In addition to the above recommendations, get used to drinking water as your main source of liquid. While it's true you obtain some of your water needs through food and other beverages, most should come from plain water, consumed between meals. Certain drinks such as coffee, tea, soda and alcohol can actually increase your need for water. So don't count these beverages as part of your water intake.

### Is Your Water Safe?

Only 1 percent of the world's water is safe to drink. Today, more people are questioning the quality of their drinking water. If you are concerned about your health, you should not just assume your water is safe to drink — you need to take active steps to find out for sure. And if there is a problem you need to correct it. Most contaminants in water fall into four categories:

- Environmental chemicals, including pesticides, herbicides and trihalomethanes, a by-product of chlorination.

- Heavy metals, including lead, copper and nitrates.

- Bacteria, including the most common coliform bacteria.

- Radiological pollution, including radon, radium and uranium.

If you're concerned about your water, the first step is to analyze it to find out what, if any, contamination exists. Once any questions about the quality of the water are answered, necessary steps to improve it can be taken more logically. The first question to ask is in regard to the source of your water. For most people, this is either a public water system or a well.

Individuals on public systems have the legal right to ask their water supplier for the results of past water tests. The supplier must also inform you of any problems, past or present, in meeting federal requirements for safety. The supplier can also tell you if your water contains chlorine or fluoride.

If your source of water comes from a well, you'll have to take the initiative and have the water tested yourself. If you've recently purchased your home, a water test should have been done before the sale. At other times, the health department may do certain tests, especially if there are local pollution problems. Deeper wells generally have less contamination than more shallow, often older, wells. Even if your area has a safe environment, many problems can come from water runoffs and chemical leaks far away from your well.

Whether you drink public or well water, another potential source of contamination is your pipes. Copper pipes may pose two different problems: the copper mineral itself, and also the lead solder. Lead solder may be seen at the joints of your pipes as a dull gray sheen. A bright, shiny color means a silver-nickel-tin product was used, which is thought to be much safer. Lead solder is not used on plastic or galvanized piping. If in doubt, a test kit available in many hardware stores can provide you with the answers.

Because lead is a serious health hazard, lead pipes were outlawed in 1986. However, in older houses (built before 1930), the plumbing may include lead pipes. These soft, dull-gray metal pipes are very dangerous, especially with soft water. Some cities, like Chicago and New York, have lead connector pipes. These are the sections that connect the city water supply with your home. The water department or city engineer should be able to tell you whether this is the case with your home.

Copper pipes can also leach the mineral into your drinking water. High copper levels occur in areas where there is soft water (sometimes referred to as a low pH or high acidity). Although not as serious as lead, excess copper can cause health problems, including disturbances of mineral balance, especially zinc, iron and manganese.

Some homes, especially in the northwestern United States, have pipes or tanks made of galvanized steel. This metal can leach cadmium, and, as with copper, this may pose health dangers.

Corrosion of pipes can also cause excess contamination. This is typical in areas where basements are damp year round. The most common source of corrosion is from the grounding of a home's electrical system. This is easy to inspect. Electrical ground wires should never be attached to your water pipes, but to a separate ground.

Although the most accurate method of analyzing your water is through a lab, observing the stains in your sink may be a clue to some contaminants. The exception is lead, which won't render any discoloration. Copper, however, will produce a blue-green stain, and iron a brown streak.

Having your water tested by a competent laboratory will remove all the guesswork regarding its safety. Samples should be taken from a frequently used source, such as the kitchen sink. A morning sample would generally have the highest levels of mineral contamination, as water sitting in the pipes all night tends to accumulate these substances. For this reason, let your water run a few seconds or more in the morning or whenever water has stayed in the pipe more than six hours, to allow that water to be discarded. If water sources in your area have been contaminated, or if several members of your household have symptoms which may relate to contaminated water (such as recurring diarrhea or vomiting) the health department will most likely do a thorough testing, perhaps free-of-charge. However, if your area has never had a problem, this service may not be available. At the least, the health department can give you names of reputable labs in your area that can test your water. These labs use Environmental Protection Agency (EPA) standards, and although some feel the EPA's ranges of normal are too conservative, at least you are ensured accurate testing. The lab may want to provide you with special collection containers, as some samples need to be properly preserved.

In some instances, such as in the case of high lead content, you may ask your doctor about testing the levels in your blood. The EPA has changed the standard for this toxic metal from 50 parts per billion (ppb) to 10 ppb when testing home water. But even at low levels, a long-term buildup in the body is always a possibility. Children are most susceptible to lead toxicity.

If you still have questions about your water, the EPA has a "Drinking Water Hotline" in Washington, D.C.: (800) 426-4791. It can provide you with a list of contaminants and the allowable levels. If you find contaminants in your water supply, there are several things you can do to remedy the problem. If the source can be corrected, such as your septic or lead pipes, this becomes an obvious priority. If the source cannot be found, a water-filtering system can usually solve your problem.

**Fluoride Safety**

The issue of fluoride and its safety is a long and complex one, and I won't attempt to cover it here. But I do want to address the use of fluoride as an additive to drinking water. I'm basically opposed to having fluoride in the water supply because it is a high-dose synthetic supplement used out of its natural environment. And, we're all forced to consume it, whether we need it or not. Instead of treating everyone with fluoridated water, an attempt should be made to target those who really need it. In the case of cavity prevention, it would be better to treat susceptible individuals than to treat entire water supplies.

More effective than fluoride in the prevention of tooth decay is maintaining proper oral pH. Some foods, mainly carbohydrates, are acid-forming. Many commercial toothpastes also make the mouth more acidic. An acidic environment in the mouth promotes tooth decay. Conversely, a more alkaline environment prevents decay. Certain foods, such as cheese, some toothpastes, and baking soda, as well as natural fats and oils will leave the mouth more alkaline. Honey is one carbohydrate food that creates an alkaline mouth chemistry and also helps to reduce dextran, a sticky substance that enables bacteria to stick to the teeth. Oral pH is especially important before bedtime. For children, a glass of apple juice or milk just before bed can promote tooth decay, and fluoride won't necessarily remedy that problem.

Despite what most people think, fluoride is no longer considered an essential nutrient. Natural fluoride is found in most foods, especially chicken, fish, seafood and tea, and it naturally occurs in most drinking water. Through a healthy diet, enough fluoride can be consumed to have a positive effect on cavity prevention. The National Institutes of Health (NIH) says tooth decay has declined sharply in recent years, even in areas without fluoridated water. British researchers also found, after studying people from eight different countries, that tooth decay was declining equally in both fluoridated and non-fluoridated areas.

Fluoride can also negatively affect other areas of the body — especially the bones. Some studies show that fluoride can substantially increase bone loss, producing bone fractures in the spine, wrist and arm. Other studies have shown that in communities that have fluoridated water, hip fractures are more common.

About half the water systems in the U.S. have fluoridated water. If you wish to avoid this water, either use bottled water or filter what comes through the tap. However, some bottled water contains fluoride (ask the company), and most water filters don't remove fluoride. The best filter for this purpose is a reverse-osmosis system.

### Filter Your Water

The first step in considering a water filter is learning what contaminants are in the water. Once you know what needs to be filtered, you can use the appropriate system. Unfortunately, there is no single water filter that will solve all your potential water problems.

Keep in mind that toxins also can enter the body through the skin or lungs when taking a shower. For example, the inhalation of trihalomethanes, a cancer-causing chemical, during showering in chlorinated water is a common problem. This can be remedied by using a system that filters all water entering your house, or by installing a water filter on your shower head.

Basically, there are four categories of water filters: activated-carbon systems, reverse-osmosis systems, ion-exchange resin filters and distillation units. Each one will filter specific contaminants.

Carbon filters, dating back to the ancient Greeks and Romans, trap contaminants as the water passes through the filter. Solid-carbon-block filters are the most effective for this process (as opposed to granular-carbon devices). Carbon filters remove most organic chemicals, such as pesticides and herbicides, chlorine, bacteria, metals (lead, iron, copper) and radon, but they do not remove minerals (so they won't soften water), nitrates, viruses and radioactive particles. Carbon filtration usually improves the taste of the water. Some carbon filters contain silver nitrate to prevent bacterial build-up; these filters may have the potential to leak silver, which is toxic. Ideally, the carbon cartridge must be replaced every six to 12 months to maintain effectiveness and normal water flow. Small carbon-filter units for water bottles are also available, making safer water possible when you are away from home.

Reverse osmosis has been used for large-scale projects, such as industrial desalination of seawater. Essentially, it's a more complex filtration system that includes carbon. Home units generally are more expensive than carbon systems when maintenance is considered. Reverse osmosis removes toxic metals and radiation contamination, except radon, but does not remove many organic chemicals. These systems tend to interfere with normal water flow (by 25 to 50 percent), and for every gallon of clean water, 6 to 8 gallons of water may be wasted.

An ion-exchange filter is a simple unit made of a resin, which filters only a few contaminants. Ion exchange removes nitrates and nitrites, toxic metals and radiation contamination, except radon. It does not remove many organic chemicals

Distillation, like carbon filtration, is also an ancient method of treating water. This is the best all-around method, as it "filters" more items than any other single device, although it is not technically a filter process. The process involves boiling the water to be treated, and capturing and cooling the steam, which gives you cleaner water. Distillation removes toxic metals and radiation contamination, except radon, and also removes minerals and thus softens the water. The downside is that it does not remove all organic chemicals and makes your water taste flat.

Manufacturers of these filtering devices can provide you with more information on which contaminants they remove as well as proper use, installation and maintenance costs. Also, it's well worth testing your water again after installing a water filter to be certain it is performing properly.

# 17 Dietary Supplements: Vitamins, Minerals and Phytonutrients

Earlier chapters discussed the importance of the macronutrients — carbohydrate, protein and fat. In this chapter I want to address two other groups of nutrients. These are the micronutrients — vitamins and minerals — and the phytonutrients, which include thousands of food compounds that not only can prevent and treat disease but also can help you achieve optimal health and fitness. Both of these groups of nutrients are used extensively as dietary supplements.

Throughout this book I have emphasized the need to eat real food and avoid processed and artificial products. The same holds true when it comes to micronutrients. It's always best to obtain vitamins and minerals from real foods, and, if you need to supplement your diet, from supplements that are made from real foods.

There are several distinctions you need to make before deciding to supplement your diet. The first thing you should determine is if you actually need a supplement. This can be accomplished in a variety of ways. Through a complete dietary analysis you can evaluate the amount of nutrients in your diet. If specific nutrients are below the recommended daily allowance (RDA), then first you are in need of dietary improvement to include or increase foods containing these nutrients. Second, you may need additional nutrients from supplements. Although following the RDA is the method most commonly used by scientists and clinicians, it is important to note that RDA levels may not be the best guide to use for nutrient intake. RDA levels don't take into account all nutrients, and many RDA levels appear inadequate for many people with certain health needs.

Another approach employed by many health-care professionals is the use of certain questionnaires such as the surveys that appear in this book. This approach is based not on nutrient levels in food but on how your body uses these nutrients. These surveys may offer clues that point to a specific nutrient, or a condition that may be associated with a nutrient. For example, sleepiness after meals, a larger waist size and frequent hunger and craving for sweets may indicate an excess intake of carbohydrates, a macronutrient. Fatigue, excess blood loss and the habit of chewing on ice may indicate the need for iron, a micronutrient. Nutritional surveys, whether self-administered or taken with the advice of a health-care professional, can be useful guides in determining your need for dietary supplements. Just be sure the survey comes from a reliable source.

**117**

If you determine that you do need to supplement for a particular nutrient, there are several things to consider. First, most dietary supplements on the market do not provide vitamins and minerals as they naturally occur in real food. Although these supplements may be labeled "natural," they are typically synthetic. They provide doses higher than nature intended, and though their chemical structures may be the same as their natural counterparts, they are really synthetic chemicals, or nutrients isolated from other key parts of the food complex in which they occur naturally. More importantly, these high-dose, synthetic and isolated supplements do not contain associated phytonutrients found in real foods. I call these supplements HSAIDS, which stands for "High-Dose Synthetic and Isolated Dietary Supplements." When consumed, HSAIDS act more like drugs than like food, thus the first major difference between HSAIDS and truly natural micronutrients.

HSAIDS are not necessarily bad, but they're not what most people think they are — equivalent to the same as the nutrient counterpart in food. The most important nutrients are those contained in foods, and if you supplement, products made from food are the best and safest choice. In some instances, such as with the careful direction of a health-care practitioner who has expertise in nutrition, HSAIDS may be required. In this case, it's usually for a relatively short period of time. It's important to understand the differences between HSAIDS and products made from real food, which technically are referred to as functional-food nutraceuticals. The differences are many and are discussed as follows.

**Biological vs. Pharmacological Effects of Supplements**
Two important distinctions between HSAIDS and truly natural supplements are whether they are made from real food, and what their function is in the human body. In general, nutrients in their natural state and natural dose have a biological effect in the body, and HSAIDS have a pharmacological effect.

Examples of dietary supplements that clearly act in more of a biological fashion include products made from vegetables, acerola, sesame oil, fish oil, nutritional yeast and garlic. These supplements provide macro-, micro- and phytonutrients with potentially great therapeutic value. They act essentially the same as when you consume real food, providing natural doses of vitamins, minerals and phytonutrients, which are essential for processes such as generating energy, regulating immunity, and controlling aging, as well as performing billions of other functions that improve health and quality of life.

Nutrients with pharmacological effects generally include HSAIDS and have actions like those of drugs rather than foods. Dietary supplements that have pharmacological effects include such common items as synthetic vitamin C (ascorbic acid), isolated vitamin E (alpha-tocopherol), and popular iron supplements. These are almost always in doses much higher than a person would normally consume during a meal or even a day's worth of food intake — even when consuming foods naturally high in these nutrients. Most supplements with pharmacological effects contain doses far exceeding what is normally present in even the best diet. Many contain doses that would take weeks of eating foods rich in these nutrients to get to the same levels — in other words, five, ten, even a hundred times normal amounts. By looking at the labels of supplements in a store or catalog, you will see that most, even those labeled "natural," contain doses much higher than you would get from real food and much higher than the RDA.

Dietary supplements that promote pharmacological activity, like most drugs, are capable of modifying body function, often in powerful ways, and are also accompanied by the risk of adverse side effects. The actions of dietary supplements with pharmacological effects can vary with individuals, and many actions are not clearly known. HSAIDS with pharmacological actions can also interfere with other nutrients, whether from the diet or other supplements, or from over-the-counter or prescription drugs.

As an example of the difference between HSAIDS and truly natural nutrients, consider vitamins C and E. Dietary sources of naturally occurring vitamin C, for example, have biological effects, acting as antioxidants and protecting DNA from oxygen damage. The dose in the best of meals may be 100 mg of vitamin C. However, the synthetic counterpart (ascorbic acid) in a dietary supplement may function differently. High doses of synthetic vitamin C, typically 500 to 1,000 mg tablets for example, can perform as an antioxidant, but can also transform to a deadly pro-oxidant — which causes excess free-radical activity and inflammation.

Another illustration of the difference between HSAIDS and truly natural nutrients is found in vitamin E. A natural dose of vitamin E is really quite small. For example, the amount of naturally occurring alpha-tocopherol in a loaf of whole-wheat bread — a relatively high source of natural vitamin E — may be only 2 to 4 IU. In contrast, the typical vitamin E dose is 400 to 800 IU, which is very high. You'd have to eat 200 loaves to reach these supplement doses. This unnatural dose of vitamin E can interfere with other more effective antioxidants and is discussed later in this chapter. There are also many potential side effects associated with HSAIDS. Consider the following:

- A cell's sensitive DNA, vital for normal function, can be damaged by consuming as little as 100 to 200 mg of synthetic vitamin C (ascorbic acid). DNA damage may be an early trigger for cancer development.

- Doses as low as 100 mg of synthetic vitamin C can act as a pro-oxidant, causing oxidative stress.

- Popular doses of vitamin C supplements can be toxic when they react with the iron in your body or iron in dietary supplements. This is because of the powerful free radicals produced by iron.

- Consuming popular doses of iron can result in excess ferritin, which has been associated with an increased risk of heart disease and liver stress. High iron intake can also produce damaging excess free radicals.

- Common preparations of copper, zinc or selenium supplements can be toxic and can even cause disease.

- Popular doses of vitamin K and B6 can be toxic.

- Consuming popular doses of vitamin A can result in bone loss and increase the risk of hip fracture in the elderly.

- Many popular HSAIDS can adversely interact with over-the-counter and prescription medications.

- In smokers, supplementation with alpha-tocopherol has been shown to increase the incidence of lung cancer.

- Consuming popular doses of beta-carotene has been shown to increase lung cancer.

- Consuming popular doses of vitamin E could increase the incidence of stroke.

In addition to knowing the potential side effects, it may be more important to understand that taking popular dietary supplements may only give you a false sense of security against the illnesses and diseases they are purported to prevent and treat. While researchers have found that consumption of fruits and vegetables decreases free-radical damage to DNA, most studies have concluded that synthetic supplements of ascorbic acid, vitamin E, or beta-carotene do not prevent DNA damage. DNA damage is one of the first steps leading to the development of cancer. Most studies also fail to show significant benefits from HSAIDS when compared to nutrients in foods.

## Natural vs. Synthetic

Consumers of dietary supplements are often confused as to what is a truly "natural" product and what is not. Many synthetic vitamins are erroneously referred to as "natural" because their chemical structures are sometimes identical or similar to the real thing. Even if you don't take a daily vitamin pill, you're probably eating some synthetic vitamins. They are added to breads, cereals and almost all packaged foods that are "fortified," as mandated by federal law since 1939.

Let's continue with vitamins C and E, two common examples of synthetic and isolated supplements, which are often sold under the "natural" label as ascorbic acid and d-alpha-tocopherol, respectively. In nature these vitamins occur with other chemical components and with associated phytonutrients as discussed later in this chapter. These supplements don't have the same function as nutrients that contain all complementary components as they occur in real food.

In addition, synthetic supplements have lower bioavailability. Using vitamin C again as an example, synthetic vitamin C is not as biologically available, and the body gets rid of it more quickly, in comparison to vitamin C in real foods. Studies have shown that vitamin C from food was 35 percent better absorbed, and excreted more slowly, than synthetic vitamin C.

Occasionally, and for short periods of time, synthetic supplements may be useful, and in fact I have recommended these to patients for many years. These synthetic products are meant as a stepping stone as you improve your diet to include the nutrients you're lacking.

## Isolated vs. the Whole-Food Complex

Some vitamins have been isolated from their whole-food complex. A common example is vitamin E, also called alpha-tocopherol. Typical doses are 400 to 800 IU. Alpha-tocopherol does not normally exist alone in nature but occurs with three other tocopherols, beta, delta and gamma, and four tocotrienols that include alpha, beta, delta and gamma. Together these seven other components of the vitamin E "complex" are more important than alpha-tocopherol alone. For example, gamma-tocopherol is commonly found in natural foods and is more effective than alpha-tocopherol as an antioxidant, especially in relation to controlling the oxidation of unsaturated fats. The common use of alpha-tocopherol supplements can be a problem since large doses of alpha-tocopherol can displace gamma-tocopherol in the body, lowering the overall oxidative protection of the vitamin E complex.

In addition, tocotrienols are powerful substances that have potent anti-cancer actions, reduce cholesterol and perform other vital tasks. Too much alpha-tocopherol can interfere with some of these functions. For example, even moderate amounts, such as 50 to 100 IU of alpha-tocopherol, can block the ability of tocotrienols to control cholesterol.

Unbalanced, high doses of alpha-tocopherol can interfere with your body chemistry in other ways too. They can have a negative effect on anti-inflammatory chemical production, cause generalized muscle weakness, lower thyroid hormone levels and slightly increased fasting triglyceride levels. Like high-dose vitamin C, alpha-tocopherol may also become a pro-oxidant — which would be counterproductive to its antioxidant function.

## The Malabsorption Syndrome

Many patients who consulted me seemed to have a need for so many nutrients. While it was tempting to urge my patients to take all these nutrients, it was clear the problem was often not the lack of nutrients but the inability of the body to absorb them. This arises most often in people under stress, which renders the intestines less effective at absorption. Any type of stress can diminish the ability of the small intestine to absorb nutrients. The stress may come from antibiotic use, even if you took the drugs months or years ago, since antibiotics destroy the natural bacteria in the large intestine, potentially changing the function of the entire intestinal tract. Whatever the stressor, the result is a low level of nutrients in the body.

This problem can often be easily remedied with a product containing both L-glutamine and a variety of acidophilus cultures. The amino acid L-glutamine is the unique energy source for the villi of the small intestine — the structures that actually absorb nutrients from food. These villi are easily damaged or destroyed under stress, by poor eating habits or by illness. An L-glutamine product that contains acidophilus cultures (such as those in yogurt) can help replace the "good bacteria" in the large intestine that may have been destroyed.

## Phytonutrients: The Real Nutrients

There are other nutritional components that may be more important than the micronutrients themselves. Many studies show that a variety of foods can protect us from cancer, heart disease and other degenerative conditions. While some assume that specific nutrients such as vitamins are responsible, it is now clear that other substances may be much more important.

These phytonutrients, or phytochemicals, are made by plants from sunlight (via photosynthesis) when grown in good-quality soil. These substances have been known in clinical nutrition for decades, and by practitioners of old for centuries. Scientists now know there are thousands of these natural chemicals that have potent therapeutic actions. Phytonutrients comprise three main groups that include phe-

| Terpenes | Phenols | Nitrogen-Containing Alkaloids |
|---|---|---|
| **Carotenoids**<br>  – alpha- and beta-carotene<br>  – lutein<br>  – lycopene<br>  – zeaxanthin<br>**Limonene**<br>**Tocopherols**<br>  – beta, delta, gamma<br>**Tocotrienols**<br>  – alpha, beta, delta, gamma | **Lignans**<br>  – sesamin<br>**Isoflavones**<br>**Flavonoids**<br>  – lutein<br>  – hesperetin<br>  – diadzein<br>  – naringin<br>  – tangeretin<br>**Tannins**<br>**Anthocyanins** | **Isothiocyanates**<br>  – sulforaphan<br>  – indol-3-carbinol<br>  – crambene<br>**Cyano-glycosides**<br>  – cocaine<br>  – nicotine<br>  – morphine<br>  – caffeine |

nols, terpenes and nitrogen-containing alkaloids. (See the table above.) Some you'll even recognize as drugs.

In studies, consumption of fruits and vegetables has been clearly shown to prevent cancer and other diseases, while classical pill-form antioxidants such as vitamin C, alpha-tocopherol and beta-carotene more often are not shown to reduce risk of disease. The differentiating factor between natural vitamin and mineral complexes and their synthetic counterparts is that truly natural supplements also contain the naturally occurring phytonutrients.

Epidemiologist John Potter of the University of Minnesota, quoted in the April 25, 1994, issue of *Newsweek*, provides us with a snapshot of the bigger scientific picture: "At almost every one of the steps along the pathway leading to cancer, there are one or more compounds in vegetables or fruit that will slow up or reverse the process." Given this, no one could, or should, conclude that taking a synthetic form of vitamin A, C or any other nutrient could be as effective as eating real foods that contain these nutrients.

The fact is, those in the natural health field have known this all along — that vitamins and minerals work best when consumed in natural doses, in the same form as they occur in natural foods. The true natural approach is to keep yourself healthy by eating real food that supplies the full spectrum of nutrients — from micronutrients to phytonutrients. Unfortunately, if you're trying to get your micronutrients from supplements, they're most likely HSAIDS — like the majority of vitamin and mineral preparations on the market. By taking these you not only risk side effects and may not be getting the whole vitamin complex, but you're missing out on the phytonutrients that accompany the natural versions.

Just remember, even though you are in charge of your body, there are times when you may need help. This is where the right professional comes in handy in helping to determine which, if any, specific nutritional supplements, dietary adjustments or lifestyle changes you may need. If you're going to use truly natural supplements, there aren't many to choose from. And, if you require a synthetic, high-dose or isolated supplement for a short period of time, seek assistance from the appropriate health-care professional.

# 18 A New Era of Dietary Supplements

Now that you understand the difference between HSAIDS and truly natural supplements, we can take a look at some different types of nutritional supplements and how they might be useful for improving your fitness and health. In this chapter I'll highlight some supplements I have found useful for my patients. At the risk of getting too close to a cookbook format, I will also give some examples of how these products are commonly used.

There are a variety of dietary supplements, functional foods and nutraceuticals on the market today — certainly enough to confuse the average consumer. Let's look at some of the definitions of these products.

The 1994 Dietary Supplement Health and Education Act (DSHEA) defines *dietary supplements* as products "intended to supplement the diet to enhance health," including vitamins, minerals, amino acids, herbs and other botanicals. It also states that a dietary supplement is "not represented as a conventional food or a sole item of a meal or the diet." Most dietary supplements fit this definition. In a 1999 edition of the journal *Science*, Steven Zeisel, M.D., defines a nutraceutical as "a diet supplement that delivers a concentrated form of a biologically active component of food in a non-food matrix in order to enhance health." This is typically a product with main ingredients that are made from "non-food" material. So a synthetic vitamin product may be considered a *nutraceutical*. In a separate category, *functional food* is defined as a food that delivers an active ingredient within the food matrix. Today there is a new era of nutritional therapy that includes the development of dietary supplements known as functional-food nutraceuticals, described below. This revolution is taking place because of the awareness of health risks of popular supplements, the realization of a lack of effectiveness of popular supplements, and the realization that food products possess powerful therapeutic capabilities.

## Functional-Food Nutraceuticals

I've been involved in research and development of functional-food nutraceuticals for many years, including the newest generation produced by MAF BioNutritionals. Functional-food nutraceuticals contain real foods containing substantial levels of compounds that have significant therapeutic actions. Most are made using certified-organic foods as raw materials to obtain the highest levels of natural nutrients without contamination from pesticides, herbicides and chemical fertilizers.

These products are made from whole foods that have been concentrated without heat by removing the water, and sometimes the fiber, to create a smaller volume. They contain amounts of therapeutic food ingredients like that of a meal or a day's worth of food. In addition to containing the specific nutrients, such as vitamin C in a vitamin C product, they also contain all the associated vitamins, minerals and phytonutrients normally found in the foods as they occur in nature. This may include hundreds if not thousands of compounds that have known therapeutic actions, or actions not yet discovered.

In the case of vitamin C, the supplement may contain citrus peel, acerola berries, beets, broccoli sprouts and other foods. Natural vitamin-C-rich foods contain many phytonutrients including limonene, tangeretin, naringin, rutin, and a whole complex of flavonoids. In order to create this kind of product, a variety of foods rich in vitamin C must be used. In this case, you will have a vitamin C content of under 100 mg.

Most companies don't produce supplements made from whole foods. It's difficult and costly to find foods dried with a low-heat process that preserves heat-sensitive nutrients, including the phytonutrients. It's even more difficult to find supplements made from certified-organic materials.

Fish oil, brewer's yeast, and other food concentrates are other examples of this category of whole-food supplements. Below are some examples of specific types of products and how a natural version may help you.

**Vitamin C Complex**

As discussed above, vitamin C in nature is accompanied by hundreds of nutrients, mostly phytonutrients that work with it to affect health and fitness. In citrus, for example, familiar compounds include rutin and hesperidin, but more potent ones include naringin, tangeretin, and limonene, just to mention some.

Vitamin C is found in relatively high concentrations in certain foods, including acerola berries, citrus peel and vegetables such as broccoli. Supplements made from real food obtain all their vitamin C from these foods, as compared to synthetically manufactured vitamin C.

Potential dangers of synthetic vitamin C in doses as low as 200 to 500 mg include DNA damage (which can be a first step in cancer production), increased risk of atherosclerosis, and its conversion to a pro-oxidant — just the opposite of a beneficial antioxidant. Oxidation puts undue stress on the immune system and increases the aging process.

In addition, vitamin C in foods is better absorbed than synthetic forms. Vitamin C from citrus, for example, is much more efficiently absorbed and utilized

than synthetic vitamin C. In addition, synthetic vitamin C is more quickly eliminated by the body than natural forms.

**Vitamin E Complex**

Vitamin E is also called alpha-tocopherol. However, as discussed in the previous
chapter, alpha-tocopherol is only one of eight compounds in the vitamin E "complex." The alpha-tocopherol fraction of the E complex does not normally exist
alone in nature but usually occurs with three other tocopherols — beta, delta,
and gamma — and four tocotrienols that include alpha, beta, delta and gamma.
Other components of the vitamin E complex can be more important than alpha-
tocopherol alone. For example, gamma-tocopherol is a very common form in
natural foods and is more effective than alpha-tocopherol as an antioxidant,
especially in relation to controlling the oxidation of unsaturated fats. Additionally, the tocotrienols are powerful substances that have potent anti-cancer actions,
reduce cholesterol and perform other vital tasks. Too much alpha-tocopherol can
interfere with some of these functions. For example, even moderate amounts of
alpha-tocopherol supplementation can block tocotrienol's important function of
controlling cholesterol.

Typical doses of alpha-tocopherol are 400 to 800 IU, a high dose which
sometimes poses a problem. At this dosage alpha-tocopherol can displace gamma-
tocopherol in the body, lowering the overall oxidative protection of the vitamin E
complex.

Unbalanced, high doses of alpha-tocopherol can interfere with your body
chemistry in other ways too. They can have a negative effect on anti-inflammatory chemical production, cause generalized muscle weakness, lower thyroid
hormone levels and slightly increase fasting triglyceride levels. Like high-dose
vitamin C, high-dose vitamin E may also become a pro-oxidant — and be counterproductive to its antioxidant function.

Almost all vitamin E supplements come in this isolated form of alpha-
tocopherol, or sometimes in a synthetic version. Some products are labeled
"mixed tocopherols" which usually is mostly alpha with very little of the other
tocopherols and no tocotrienols.

**Immune-System Support**

Immune-system support is the most important role of antioxidants. Immune support provides maximum protection against the onset of cancer and other chronic
disease. Natural forms of vitamin C and E are just two of these disease-fighting
substances. Also vital for immune-system support are other antioxidants or nutri-

ents which promote antioxidant activity, the most powerful being lipoic acid, cysteine (sometimes in the form of N-acetyl-cysteine) and sulforaphan, a sulfur compound in cruciferous vegetables such as broccoli, kale, Brussels sprouts and cabbage. Two- to three-day-old broccoli sprouts (before their leaves turn green) have the highest levels of sulforaphan. Traditional antioxidant supplements are void of these naturally occurring powerful compounds. Both alpha-tocotrienol and gamma-tocopherol are also more powerful antioxidants than either alpha-tocopherol or vitamin C.

In addition, phytonutrients such as limonene, naringin and tangeretin support the process of apoptosis — a reaction that triggers the death of cancer cells. These compounds are found in the skins of citrus fruits.

The full spectrum of carotenoids, including lycopene, are also key elements in foods that make up an ideal supplement to support immune function, along with turmeric and ginger.

One of the keys to improving immune function is to stimulate the production of glutathione. This is accomplished with a number of the above compounds, especially lipoic acid, cysteine and sulforaphan. A variety of other nutrients, such as riboflavin, zinc and selenium, are also important in supporting all these compounds in their immune-support role.

**Whole-Food Multiple Supplements**

The natural counterpart to the synthetic multiple vitamin is the whole-food multiple-vitamin/mineral supplement made from real foods. Ingredients for these products include a variety of vegetables such as kale, Brussels sprouts, beets, carrots, broccoli, spinach and parsley; fruits such as citrus and berries; and natural nutritional yeasts which contain the B vitamins. These supplements contain a food dose of all the vitamins, minerals and phytonutrients. Since they're made from real food, they probably contain nutrients not yet discovered!

**Omega-3 Fats**

In my practice, I found through dietary analysis that significant numbers of patients were deficient in omega-3 fats. It has been estimated that more than 50 million people in the United States are affected by essential-fatty-acid imbalance. In the chapters on fats, we learned that too little series 3 eicosanoids produced from omega-3 fats can contribute to many health problems.

Omega-3 oils are most useful in reducing the condition of chronic inflammation. Fish oil contains both EPA and DHA, vital for many aspects of optimal health and fitness, especially combating inflammation. A variety of other foods complement this task, including ginger, garlic, turmeric, citrus peel and sesame oil. The best omega-3 supplement is Nature's Dose™ Infla-min Anti-Inflammatory Complex, which contains all these powerful foods. If you wish to supplement with fish oil, keep these points in mind:

- Make sure the oil has been tested for oxidation.

- Make sure the oil has been tested for heavy metals and other potential toxins found in the oceans. A good guide is to use fish oil that states it has "0" cholesterol. Many state levels of only 2 or 4 mg of cholesterol, but this infers they may not have been cleaned of potential toxins.

- If you eat cold-water ocean fish such as salmon and tuna to provide omega-3 fats, don't cook the fish too much — less is best since the oils are easily damaged by heat. Much of the fish today is raised in fish farms and these fish contain less EPA.

For those who don't want to take fish oil as a source of omega-3, flaxseed oil is an option. However, there are two important factors to consider. Since flaxseed oil is extremely susceptible to oxidation when exposed to air or heat, it is best to purchase it in capsules. Without specific nutrients, including vitamins C, B6, niacin, and the minerals magnesium and zinc, flax oil can't be converted to EPA required to be therapeutic in the body and is simply stored as fat. Even if all necessary co-factors are present, some sources say every gram of EPA requires 11 grams of omega-3 from vegetable sources.

The dose for omega-3 fat supplementation is highly individual, and is best determined through a dietary analysis, and by observing how much you require to control signs and symptoms of inflammation if any exist. Very healthy individuals may need to take 1 to 3 capsules per day, but individuals in poor health with high levels of inflammation may need to take from 10 to 16 omega-3 capsules daily until symptoms subside. If you use flax instead of fish, more may be required. If you are unsure of whether you have inflammation, the best way to evaluate its presence is a blood test for C-reactive protein levels.

**Black-Currant-Seed Oil**
Black-currant-seed yields a high-quality omega-6 oil containing gamma-linolenic acid (GLA) which is converted to the series 1 anti-inflammatory eicosanoids. People with allergies, especially in the spring when natural series 1 eicosanoid levels are low, often need this supplement. GLA is also essential for carrying calcium to muscle

**129**

and bone cells. Without it, the calcium in your diet won't be as useful and will often simply be stored as calcium deposits. Borage oil and evening primrose oil also contain GLA.

It's important when taking any product containing GLA to also take raw sesame-seed oil. This contains a phytonutrient called sesamin which prevents GLA from ultimately converting to arachidonic acid, which promotes inflammation. Both sesame and all the GLA-containing oils are very sensitive to oxygen, and should be purchased in capsule form.

**Vitamin B Complex**
Vitamins were named in alphabetical order as they were discovered — first A, followed by B, then C. Only after this process was begun was it realized that vitamin B contained a number of similar but distinct compounds, which ultimately were named B1, B2, etc. There is now a large group of vitamins in this category, referred to as the "B complex." However, the various B vitamins are as different from each other as they are from other, non-B vitamins. They share only one strong similarity — they are all water-soluble. This has little to do with anything other than in knowing they are not stored for long periods in the body as are the fat-soluble vitamins. The use of nutritional yeast is perhaps the best source of the B vitamins in supplements. In almost all supplements however, synthetic B vitamins are used.

Today, some of the B vitamins are referred to as they were traditionally, by number (such as B6), and others are referred to by name (such as niacin). In this book I will follow this common method. Below is a very brief synopsis of some of the important features of certain B vitamins. But realize that a complete discussion of just the B vitamins and how they impact health and fitness would fill many chapters.

Vitamin B1 (thiamin) and B2 (riboflavin) are sometimes used separately as their actions in the body are uniquely different. For example, athletes tend to use more vitamin B1 because intense physical activity can produce so much lactic acid; B1 is very important in reducing lactic acid. Some people need both B1 and B2. This is especially true in the elderly, those on certain medications and those with heart problems. Like most nutrients, B1 is best taken in lower doses like those found in food. In fact, lower doses are as effective as higher ones, and doses above 2.5 to 5 mg are mostly unabsorbed.

Vitamin B6 (pyridoxine) and niacin (B3) are important in many bodily functions, but especially in the conversion of omega-6 and -3 fats to their respective anti-inflammatory eicosanoids.

Folic acid and vitamin B12 are key nutrients for protecting the heart and brain against conditions such as heart disease and Alzheimer's. When these nutrients are in short supply, levels of homocysteine rise, which also raises the risk of these diseases. These nutrients are also important for healthy blood and the ability of the body to carry sufficient oxygen to all its cells. Folic acid is especially important for maintenance and repair of the intestines, and for many other functions.

There are really a variety of folic-acid compounds in nature, in different natural-folate forms. Only folic acid from foods and from supplements made from foods contains the entire complex of many naturally occurring folates. However, the folic acid contained in virtually all supplements, a synthetic form, does not occur in nature. And unfortunately, a significant number of people are not able to absorb the popular synthetic folic acid. These people must rely on natural sources. Folate-rich foods include spinach, lettuce, kale and other leafy vegetables, with fruit also containing some of the valuable forms.

### Calcium

Few people in industrialized societies have true calcium deficiencies, regardless of what the advertisements tell us. The bigger problem is that most people are unable to utilize the calcium they already have in their bodies. Poor calcium metabolism, rather than deficiency, is almost at epidemic proportions. The end result is that not enough calcium gets into the cells, including the bones, muscles and other tissues, with the remaining excess calcium depositing in the joints, tendons, ligaments or even the kidneys as stones.

In order for your body to properly metabolize calcium, you must first consume enough calcium-rich foods; this is easily done without supplementation through good dietary practices that include lots of vegetables and fish. Consider the high amounts of calcium in the following single servings of non-dairy foods:

| | | | |
|---|---|---|---|
| Salmon | .225 mg | Sardines | .115 mg |
| Soybeans | .175 mg | Almonds | .100 mg |
| Seaweed | .140 mg | Rainbow trout | .100 mg |
| Spinach | .135 mg | Green beans | .100 mg |
| Collards | .125 mg | | |

Unfortunately, many people won't eat enough of these calcium-rich foods and for them supplementation may be necessary.

But just consuming calcium is only the first step. It must then be absorbed from the foods or supplements. In the case of many types of supplements, absorbability is poor. This is due to both the type (e.g., calcium carbonate products are poorly absorbed), and dose, as discussed in the following paragraph. And finally, calcium must be brought from the blood into the bone or muscle. Calcium metabolism is regulated by the hormonal system. In general, the amount of calcium intake need not be high, whether in the diet or supplements, to produce the desired effects, such as strong bones. Rather, it's the efficiency with which the body uses this important mineral that counts.

Absorption is the first step to utilizing calcium in the body. In general, small amounts are absorbed better than larger amounts, whether from food or supplements. If a small amount of calcium is present in the intestine, 70 percent may be absorbed, for example, while a larger amount of calcium may have only a 30 percent absorption rate. If you're taking calcium supplements, it may be best to take a lower dose several times a day rather than a large dose once daily. Vitamin D production, stimulated by sunshine, is also an important factor for calcium absorption as well as cancer prevention as discussed in chapter 34.

Vegetables, which contain smaller amounts of calcium, may be a better source than milk, which contains large amounts of the mineral. Not only does milk have a larger amount of calcium, but its phosphorus content reduces calcium absorption. So in some situations, a serving of broccoli may result in more calcium getting into the body than a serving of milk.

The stomach's natural hydrochloric acid is also very important in making calcium more absorbable. Neutralizing stomach acid has a negative effect on calcium absorption, and a serious impact on digestion and absorption of all nutrients. Once absorbed, calcium is utilized best when the body is in a slightly acidic state. Otherwise, calcium that is absorbed may be more easily deposited in joints, muscles or arteries rather than inside the cells where it's needed. The cells that are calcium-starved cause symptoms such as muscle tightness and irritability, identical to those of calcium deficiency. Morning stiffness, which loosens up only after moving around for a while, is one of the most common symptoms of this calcium problem. Signs of an advanced problem include so-called bone spurs (a deposit of calcium in the ligament) or kidney stones. Rather than needing more calcium, these people need more acidity. Two teaspoons daily of apple-cider vinegar may help maintain the proper pH to help calcium work properly. This can be taken as part of your salad dressing, or even mixed into a 4-ounce glass of water. Supplements such as betaine hydrochloride (see below) also help promote the acidity necessary for calcium absorption.

Cold sores on the lip, cheek and tongue usually indicate a need for calcium, as do tight muscles, and difficulty falling asleep when you first go to bed. Too much yard work in the spring, a first game of tennis in years, or an increase in exercise can cause muscle soreness, which can respond well to calcium, as do menstrual cramps (a form of muscle cramp), itchy skin and hives.

Furthermore, there are substances that can deplete calcium. Excess carbohydrates often contain too much fiber and phytic acid, which can block calcium absorption. Caffeine reduces calcium levels in blood. Phosphorus can be the most detrimental, pulling calcium out of bones and muscles. Most soft drinks contain large amounts of phosphorus — and the people who drink them risk significant calcium loss from their teeth and bones.

Calcium is part of the body's complex chemical makeup. As such, it must be balanced with all other nutrients, especially magnesium. Too much calcium can cause a magnesium deficiency. Magnesium is necessary for most enzymes to work, including the ones important for fat metabolism. One of the best calcium materials for supplements is bone meal, discussed later in this chapter.

### Some Facts and Myths of Osteoporosis

Osteoporosis is usually a multifactorial problem, meaning there's hardly ever just one cause. We know that a lack of calcium is usually not the cause, nor is low estrogen. Methods that are effective in treating or preventing osteoporosis in one person may have very different results in someone else. Osteoporosis may not be as much of a problem as it has been made into. As Susan Brown, Ph.D., author of *Better Bones, Better Body* (Keats Publishing, New Canaan, Conn., 1996) emphasizes:

- Osteoporosis itself doesn't cause bone fractures; half of those with osteoporosis never get fractures.

- Severely osteoporotic vertebrae are strong enough to withstand five times the normal weight bearing.

- Menopause does not, per se, cause osteoporosis, and only 15 percent of a woman's bones are affected by estrogen.

- Zinc and magnesium may be as important as calcium for bones.

- Up to 80 percent of all hip-fracture patients may have a vitamin D deficiency.

### Iron

Iron is an important nutrient for all areas of the body, especially the blood and the aerobic muscles. It's also important in the brain and nervous system; it aids in the production of neurotransmitters and other brain chemicals, and is in the protective covering of nerves.

It is possible to have normal iron in the blood but too little in the muscles, causing muscle dysfunction. Since aerobic muscle burns fat, a person with low muscle iron may have trouble burning fat. If supplements are necessary, a relatively low daily dose, such as 10 mg, for a month or two may be enough. If you have a continuous need for iron, something more important may be missing. Taking iron for long periods, in small or large amounts, may be harmful.

Iron is efficiently recycled in the body, with some loss occurring through sweating during exercise, or for women, through menstruation. Excess iron loss or decreased intake may produce a serious deficiency.

On the other extreme, toxic amounts of iron may be deposited in the liver and spleen, resulting in cirrhosis of the liver or diabetes. Excess iron is also associated with certain neurological problems including Alzheimer's and Parkinson's disease, and multiple sclerosis. Since the early 1980s, scientists have known of important relationships between high levels of stored iron and heart disease. Excess iron, even moderate amounts, may even prove to be a more significant risk factor for heart disease than excess cholesterol.

When the body has enough iron for normal use, the remainder is stored in the form of ferritin. Evidence shows that ferritin may promote the formation of free radicals. These may injure cells lining the arteries and damage heart muscle, as well as increase the level of LDL, the so-called bad cholesterol.

The marketing of iron to treat fatigue ("iron-poor, tired blood") may be one reason for excess accumulation of iron in some people, as iron supplements are still very popular. Almost all multiple-vitamin/mineral preparations contain too much of it, and many foods are fortified with iron. Certainly, if you are iron deficient, taking an iron supplement is necessary. But without knowing whether it's needed, traditional iron supplementation should be avoided.

If a blood test for ferritin shows you have too much stored iron, the first thing to do is assess whether you are consuming too much. Often, excess iron stores are the result of an accumulation of iron over several years. The use of iron cookware also can contribute to high iron stores. In some situations, the body's metabolism may not be functioning properly, resulting in excess ferritin. Donating blood may be one way to help reduce excess iron stores.

## Choline

This nutrient is critical for proper fat metabolism, preventing the deposit of fat in the liver, and is associated with adrenal-gland and heart function. Choline is also very important in brain function where acetylcholine synthesis is vital. Egg yolks, fish and wheat germ are excellent sources of choline in the diet.

A common indication for the need for choline supplementation is asthma. Wheezing, coughing from bronchial spasm, and excessive mucous production during exercise has been termed "exercise-induced asthma" (although it occurs more in those who don't exercise) and is typically associated with a need for choline. Normally, the body's response to activity or exercise is to dilate the airway passages to allow for better air passage. With exercised-induced asthma, this dilation is followed by excess narrowing of the air passages. Choline can help the nervous system control proper bronchial action.

### Case History

*Roy was a slim, 44-year-old construction worker who wanted to "run with the guys" after work, though he could run with them for only about 15 minutes due to his severe asthmatic reactions. This was due in part to the stress of running at too high a heart rate without proper training, but also a need for choline. After two weeks of taking choline, his symptoms were gone. Eighteen months later, after improving his aerobic system and eating eggs daily to keep his choline intake adequate, Roy qualified for and competed in the world masters' track and field meet in Australia, where he won a box full of medals.*

## Organ and Gland Products

Most people who take nutritional supplements are familiar with the many animal concentrates available: liver, thymus and kidney as well as other organ and gland tissues. Clinically it is known that these products can be a great help to your health, though scientists still don't agree on why they work. Organ and gland "meats" have been a delicacy for humans throughout history, and only recently have we looked askance at them.

Products containing thymus may be especially helpful for the immune system. Human thymus function gradually diminishes with age, resulting in the alteration of T-cell functions in the elderly. However, the loss of function can be reversed. Studies show bovine thymus from supplements remains active when administered orally to humans. Other studies show thymus has been used successfully for the treatment of food allergies and respiratory infections, and has been shown to regulate maturation of human T-cells, which improve immune function.

Bone meal is one of the best natural materials for calcium supplementation. In addition to providing all the nutrients normally found in bone, this supplement can help ligament, tendon and muscle problems, including sprains, strains, and other mechanical injuries. It can also be used for tooth problems, especially those related to bone loss.

Many other animal products can be found in dietary supplements. These include heart, adrenal gland, pancreas, thyroid and brain. They should be free of hormones and dried without heat to preserve the vital nutrients, but made safe from harmful bacteria or virus. To be safe, look for certified-organic products to be sure the source animals had not been fed animal parts or exposed to other animals that may have been sick.

### Intestinal Support

The amino acid L-glutamine and a variety of "friendly" bacterial cultures, like those found in yogurt, are two products important for intestinal function. L-glutamine helps the intestine absorb nutrients by improving the function of the villi — tiny finger-like projections in the intestine that pull nutrients out of food to bring into the blood. This amino acid reduces intestinal distress, improves immunity, and can protect the delicate intestines from the dangers of aspirin and other harmful chemicals. L-glutamine also has anti-inflammatory functions. With such names as lactobacillus acidophilus and salivarius, bifidobacterium bifidum, and streptococcus thermophilus, "friendly" bacteria in supplement form are very helpful if you ever need to take an antibiotic, which can destroy your friendly bacteria. This is also a problem in people with many types of intestinal problems, especially due to stress or when traveling. The intestinal bacteria are vital to overall health, helping to regulate intestinal function, including nutrient absorption, production of vitamins and elimination of waste and excess cholesterol. As noted previously, folic acid is also important for intestinal function.

### Betaine Hydrochloride

Contrary to popular belief, most people with upset stomachs have too little, rather than too much, stomach acid. Even those whose stomachs feel fine can have problems. Stress and aging are the two most common reasons for reduction of natural hydrochloric acid in the stomach, which is vital for a number of important aspects of health. This natural acid is required for the proper digestion of foods, especially proteins. A lack of natural stomach acid can result not only in impaired protein absorption, but also deficiencies in calcium, vitamin B12, iron and zinc. Stomach acid also plays a significant role in intestinal function, as well as protection against infections, including Candida, and diseases such as rheumatoid arthritis and stomach cancer. Betaine hydrochloride, the salt of hydrochloric acid that turns into the same natural stomach acid, can be taken to increase natural stomach acid. I recommend taking it after meals and snacks until intestinal function returns to normal. In some people a long-term need for betaine hydrochloride exists.

## Skin Care

The omega-6 fat GLA is perhaps the best remedy for skin problems. Breaking open a gel cap of black-currant-seed oil and rubbing it into the skin is a great remedy for dry skin, wrinkles, or even the most stubborn skin problems, as good if not better than all the expensive skin remedies on the market. It's also good for burns, including sunburn, but only after the skin has been thoroughly cooled.

Shea butter is a unique skin-care product made from an African nut extract (similar to a coconut) and has been used for centuries as a beauty product. European studies have shown that shea butter is remarkably active against skin blemishes and irritation. It's also useful as a daily hand, face or body ointment. As a moisturizer, it is helpful against the damaging effects of the sun and also helps maintain the skin's elasticity. Look for 100 percent shea butter with no fragrance or other artificial ingredients.

For sun protection, a number of nutritional substances can be effective. These are nutrients you can take internally rather than topically as a sunscreen. Your body uses up a number of substances rapidly after sun exposure. These include folic acid, beta-carotene and lycopene. Studies show that tocotrienols help protect the skin directly, and limonene can protect against skin cancer. Any of the antioxidants will also help with sun exposure since increased free radicals are one harmful effect of the sun. In addition, omega-3 fats, especially fish oil, help protect the skin during sun exposure. But take omega-3 oils at least a week or two before being in the sun, or take them regularly if you're often in the sun.

Ideally, all supplements should be chewed, not just swallowed — just like when you're eating any other real food. Tasting your supplements improves their function in your body, due to the "cephalic phase" of digestion. The only exception is products containing betaine hydrochloride. In general, supplements are best taken with meals, although in many cases it does not matter since real food products such as functional-food nutraceuticals are in themselves real food. So taking them any time, between, before, during or after meals can be effective. Again, an exception is betaine hydrochloride, which should always be taken after meals. These non-prescription supplements are available in health-food stores and from nutrition-oriented health-care professionals.

# 19 Snacking Your Way to Health

Thus far we've discussed what to eat, and how much of what to eat. But there's yet another component to healthy eating habits that can make a positive difference in your health — how often you eat. Specifically, eating more frequently, or snacking between major meals, can improve your health in many ways. In fact, perhaps no other single dietary habit can make a more positive difference in your health than snacking.

In our society, snacks are generally seen as an unhealthful addition of unwanted calories and fat, and something to avoid. This can be quite true if you snack on junk food such as candy bars, snack cakes, chips and crackers that are full of sugar, refined carbohydrates and unhealthy fats. Between-meal binges on junk foods like these can be devastating to your health. But healthy, real-food snacks that contain balanced macronutrients have many health benefits and can help provide your mind and body with a continuous supply of the fuel necessary for optimal human performance. Scientific and medical studies also show that healthy snacking can help you control blood-sugar levels, improve metabolism, reduce stress and cholesterol, burn more body fat and increase energy levels.

**Keep It Small, Keep It Real**
A healthy snack is just a small meal. The key to healthful snacking is to reduce the amount of food eaten at regular meals, and distribute this nutritional wealth throughout the day. I call snacks "mini-meals." And truly that's the approach you want to take. Eat five or six smaller meals that add up to the same amount of food that you would normally consume in a typical three-meal-a-day routine. The ideal plan is to start the day with a good balanced breakfast that includes an adequate serving of quality protein. For example, eggs and whole-grain toast, or plain yogurt and fruit can get your day off to a good start. Skipping breakfast may be one of the worst nutritional bad habits, but worse yet is eating a high-carbohydrate breakfast of cereal or a bagel, which can be counterproductive, negating all the effects of this more healthy style of eating. From breakfast on, plan to eat every two to four hours. A schedule that works well for many people is a good breakfast, followed by a snack at 10 a.m., lunch at noon, another snack at 2 or 3 p.m., a light dinner, and if necessary a snack later in the evening. Healthy snacks can be almost anything you like, just as long as they are made from real, healthy food. For many people, snacks, like regular meals, should con-

tain protein. Experiment to discover how much food you need and which types work best. Some people may need to eat much larger snacks but others can get by on minimal amounts. Avoid junk food and high-carbohydrate snacks. Ideally, snacks should be just like any meal, containing a proper balance of carbohydrate, protein and fat. Use the guidelines you have learned in previous chapters to help you determine the macronutrient balance of your snacks just like you would any other meals. If this is too complicated or not always practical to compute for all your snacks, a two-to-one ratio of carbohydrate to protein sometimes works as a general guideline.

Snacks should also supply adequate vitamins, minerals and phytonutrients — from the foods themselves. Therefore do not overlook fruits and vegetables when choosing snacks. A vegetable snack can be a stick of raw celery stuffed with almond butter, or a bowl of leftover chicken-vegetable soup. Similarly a fruit-based snack can be an apple with a handful of almonds, or berries blended with plain yogurt in a smoothie. Be creative. Seek out variety in your snacks just as you would with other meals.

It is important to keep a variety of healthful snack foods on hand at all times, so make plans for your snacking habits on your next visit to the grocery store. Leftovers from healthy meals make great snacks, so plan your meals for extras. Other examples of healthful snacks include raw almonds or a chunk of cheese with a piece of fruit, raw almond butter with fresh apple or pear slices, or a mixed-vegetable salad with hard-boiled eggs, meat or fish. Phil's Bars™ and Alma bars™ are also healthful, real-food snacks that you can take with you on the road.

### The Benefits of Healthy Snacking

Although this approach is different from the way you may be accustomed to eating, you will find it quickly suppresses cravings, especially for junk foods, improves physical and mental energy, and stimulates weight loss. Inside your body something else will happen — your metabolism will change. Since snacking stabilizes blood sugar and prompts your body to produce less insulin, your body will store less fat and use more of it to fuel all your daily activities from work to play. Many people find that they have much more energy when following a program of healthy snacking.

Controlling insulin through healthy snacking can also help your body counteract the harmful effects of daily stress. This reduced stress brings about many health advantages, including less production of the adrenal hormone cortisol, which, like insulin, also prompts your body to store fat. Cortisol also can disrupt sleep patterns, and adrenal stress is a common thread in people who wake during the middle of the night. If left unchecked, adrenal stress is the first in a series of functional problems that can lead to disease, as discussed in chapter 31. Snacking also helps to reduce cholesterol. A recent long-term study published in the *British Medical Journal* showed that eating more frequently lowers blood cholesterol, specifically LDL, known as the "bad" cholesterol. This confirms results of other earlier studies showing the effect of snacking on lowering cholesterol. In addition, studies show a staggering 30 percent increase in heart disease in those eating three meals or less per day.

While snacking has received a bad rap over the years, experts now agree that it was the type of food, not the frequency of eating, that caused problems. In addition, just piling on the calories by adding snacks to an already unhealthy diet is clearly dangerous. Now we know that eating healthy, balanced snacks throughout the day can help you improve your health in many ways.

# 20 Eat, Drink and Be Merry

Food is inextricably linked to the human psyche. Early humans knew they had to eat to survive and so food was a primary focus. In times of plenitude, food became associated with festivity. Today, humans are really not any different, but the types of foods and the amounts have changed radically. In this culture every day is a day of plenitude for most, and unfortunately junk food is at the top of the menu. The furious pace of day-to-day life causes many to resort to highly processed fast food and convenience food. What's more, people have learned to equate sweets with everything from love to reward, giving candy for Valentine's Day and telling children they can't have dessert until they finish their vegetables. So while food is still at the forefront of the thought process, for most it's a process that has gone awry.

Food should be festive — among the top pleasures in life is a delicious, satisfying and healthy meal. Too many people have lost their natural inclination for this sensation. We should eat, drink and be merry if we want to live a long and healthy life. That does not mean we should abuse food and drink. Instead we should know what and how much to eat and drink, and our merriness should be genuine.

At one time, people instinctively knew what to eat. Today, large corporations spend billions of dollars telling us what we're hungry for. And it works. How many times have you been watching a commercial on TV and suddenly had an intense craving for whatever was being advertised? We can't choose our meals and snacks by what looks good in a TV commercial — that is, not if we want to be healthy and fit.

Previous chapters have set the table for you to change, modify or fine-tune your current eating style. These guidelines are relatively simple, although there seems to be many of them. Other guidelines require more explanation. In this chapter are some tips for shopping, food preparation and eating.

## Shopping for Health

The most important first step you can take for better dietary habits is to learn to properly shop for the food items that will bring about the greatest health. Bad food has less of a chance of getting into your body if it never gets into your grocery cart. With a little thought, planning and effort, you can make sure only healthy items get into your cart and your body.

Begin planning your shopping trip before you leave home. Never shop or make a shopping list when you are hungry because you will tend to buy more junk including sweets. Instead, have a snack, make a list and decide where you will shop. Years ago people shopped at different stores for different foods. But in these days of "one-stop shopping," it isn't always possible or convenient. If you are limited to one stop, pick the store that reliably has the most items on your list. Many cities now have health-food supermarkets, and many of the larger chain groceries now carry higher-quality foods, such as organic produce.

In most grocery stores, you will find that most of the real-food items are stocked on the store's perimeter. While making this loop, try to buy as few items in packages as possible. If you do buy items in packages, always be sure to read the label and study the list of ingredients and nutritional facts. If the item contains anything that does not promote health, it belongs back on the shelf and not in your cart. In addition, choose organic items when available. Stick to your list. Remembering everything on it will keep you focused and help you avoid such dietary pitfalls as the fresh-baked French bread (full of refined white flour and fake vitamins) that grocers place strategically and aromatically at the ends of store aisles.

Your most important stop on the store perimeter is the produce section. Choose a variety of fresh greens and vegetables for salads and cooking. Avoid starchy potatoes and corn. Once again, look for organic produce, especially if you are buying spinach or celery, as these crops are often heavily sprayed and can retain high pesticide residues. Also in the produce section are fresh fruits. Minimize the high-glycemic fruits such as bananas and watermelon, and instead choose fiber-rich apples and grapefruits, and phytonutrient-rich berries.

Next stop is the meat section. Seek out natural or organic grass-fed beef, pork and lamb, free-range poultry and wild-caught ocean fish. These more-natural meats can be found in many supermarkets and health-food groceries. If you can't find these types of meats in stores, many are available by mail order.

Bakeries are usually located on the store perimeter. If you stop at the bakery, be especially careful to choose items made entirely from whole grains, such as sprouted-grain or 100 percent whole-wheat bread. Read labels carefully to make sure that bakery items do not contain white flour, sugar or hydrogenated oils. Don't even consider doughnuts! (See the sidebar on doughnuts, and you'll be convinced.)

Also on the outer edge of the grocery you will find the dairy section. If you must buy milk, consider goat milk, which is closer in composition to human milk than cow milk, as discussed later in this chapter. Cream, butter, cottage cheese and fully cultured yogurt and cheese contain little or no lactose, a sugar that is difficult for many people to digest. Read the nutritional facts on these dairy products — carbohydrates and sugars should be very low. When buying high-fat dairy products look for organic items, since toxins such as pesticides and hormones often bind to the fat in dairy products.

Near the dairy section are the eggs. Most stores now carry eggs from free-range hens, and many also carry organic eggs. They cost a little more but are still a protein bargain.

If you stick to the perimeter of the store, you'll find that you only rarely need venture up an aisle. Usually the only food items you'll need up the aisles are extra-virgin olive oil, raw unfiltered honey, beans, nuts, nut butters, spices and sea salt.

## Tips for Healthy Cooking

How you cook your food can be just as important as how you select it, since even the healthiest ingredients can be destroyed through improper kitchen practices. The biggest problems are overcooking, using too-high heat, and overheating certain types of oils. Following are some guidelines that can help make your work in the kitchen become a work of health.

### Deadly Doughnuts

Love the taste of doughnuts? If you want to be healthy you better get over it. Even though some are "cholesterol-free," these crispy items are one junk food to avoid. Their bad ingredients include trans fats, sugar, refined flour, artificial flavors and colors, and many other chemicals with names you can't pronounce.

But there's more danger — the ingredients tell nothing of what really gives doughnuts their unique crispy flavor. Most doughnut makers buy oil that other fast-food operations have already used to fry their products. This tired oil often has been used to fry other foods for weeks. The intense heat breaks down the oil and turns some of it to soap. This combination gives doughnuts their special crispy taste and texture, something that fresh oil fails to do. There are many other flour products made with used oil out there as well, so beware.

The main problem is that these oils — overcooked trans fats — can adversely affect the delicate balance of fats in your body, producing too many cancer-promoting prostaglandins. Along the way, inflammation, increased blood pressure and other problems can be triggered too. Even just one doughnut contains enough of these dangerous fats to remain in the body and trigger unhealthy actions for months.

145

The worst method for cooking anything is deep-fat or high-heat frying, especially using vegetable oils. While many healthy foods may be lightly sautéed in butter or olive oil, deep-frying overheats the oil and can be deadly. In addition, the high heat may destroy other nutrients in the food itself.

Meats, fish and poultry can be grilled, roasted or cooked in their own juices with sea salt. Less oil or butter is needed for pan-cooking meats because they often contain sufficient fats. Additionally, most people overcook meats and destroy some of the valuable nutrients. It's also important to not use too-high heat for too long. For instance when grilling a steak, remember to turn it every minute or so to prevent the excess formation of chemicals that can be harmful to your health. This goes for vegetables as well — if using high heat remember to turn them often.

Vegetables can be steamed, stir-fried in olive oil, roasted, baked or grilled. Cook vegetables minimally to avoid destroying vitamins and phytonutrients — they also taste better when not overcooked. If boiling or steaming, use as little water as possible to avoid leaching of nutrients.

Eggs can be soft- or hard-boiled, or cooked sunny-side up, over-easy, poached or lightly scrambled. Use low heat to avoid "tough" or rubbery eggs.

If using oils for cooking it's important to remember that all oils contain varying ratios of monounsaturated, saturated and polyunsaturated fats. Monounsaturated and saturated fats are not sensitive to heat, but polyunsaturated oils are very prone to oxidizing when exposed to heat. This oxidation produces free

### Rediscovering Lard

You've probably been programmed to believe that the absolute "worst" fat you can consume is lard. Well, that's a commonly held belief, but consider the facts. Many people are surprised to learn that compared to butter, lard contains more heart-healthy monounsaturated fat, and less saturated fat and cholesterol.

LARD

A tablespoon of lowly lard contains 5.7 grams of monounsaturated fat compared to 3.3 for butter. Lard weighs in at 5 grams of saturated fat compared to 7.1 for butter. And lard contains less than half the cholesterol of butter — 12.1 mg compared to 31 mg. Lard also contains less heat-sensitive polyunsaturated fat than olive oil — 1.4 grams compared to 2.

For these reasons, lard may be a better choice for cooking than butter or olive oil. It is preferred by many chefs for its flavor and its ability to withstand heat. And it's inexpensive, too. A pound can cost less than 50 cents.

radicals, which are related to many health problems. Butter is one of the safest oils for cooking, as it contains a low amount of polyunsaturated fat, only 4 percent. Olive oil can also be used for cooking but its polyunsaturated content is a little higher at 9 percent. This is still much better than, for instance, peanut oil, which contains 33 percent polyunsaturated, or worse yet, safflower oil at 77 percent. As strange as it may sound, another fat you may consider is lard, which contrary to popular belief may be a healthier choice for cooking than butter.

## Some Tips for Eating

The human digestive system requires that food be chewed well before it is swallowed. It's extremely important to remember to sufficiently chew your food. Chickens have a gizzard, which grinds their food, so they just swallow their food whole. The way some people eat, you'd think they have a gizzard too! Chewing does more than chop the food into smaller pieces. It's the beginning of the very important first stage of digestion, especially for carbohydrates. Chewing and mixing saliva with your food triggers reactions in the brain, which sends messages to the rest of the body, preparing it to process and utilize the food. Many digestive-related problems can be greatly improved, if not eliminated, by properly chewing food.

Meals should be eaten in a relaxed environment. This means not while working, getting the kids ready for school or arguing about money. Get away from your stress, get off your feet, and relax. This allows the digestive system to function most efficiently. Enjoying a glass of wine with a meal may help promote this relaxation, as discussed later in this chapter.

Eat some raw food at each meal — it may help digestion and your body's response to the meal. Examples of raw additions include avocado, raw nuts, soft-cooked eggs (raw yolk), and the traditional vegetables and fruits. Certain natural-food supplements also contain foods not processed at high temperatures and can be considered "raw."

Once you develop your natural intuition, which will come in time, you'll know when you're hungry and when you're full. This will keep you from over-eating and over-taxing your system.

The work of the noted Russian physiologist Ivan Pavlov also should be acknowledged when considering eating habits. Pavlov is best known for experiments with ringing bells and salivating dogs. But more importantly, he was also engaged in some very important research about eating habits. Pavlov found that different food groups evoked very different reactions from the digestive tract. He divided these foods into four basic groups:

• Concentrated protein such as meats, fish, cheese and eggs

- Concentrated carbohydrates such as breads, potatoes, sugar-containing foods and fruits

- Fat

- Milk

These foods, he said, were digested by the body in very different ways, requiring different chemical reactions and digesting at very different rates. Combining any two of these food groups, especially the first two, could result in digestive stress, poor digestion, and poor absorption of nutrients.

Individuals have many different responses to various foods and combinations of foods. If you have digestive problems, including excess gas production, intestinal irritation or poor nutrient absorption, you may wish to follow Pavlov's advice and avoid mixing these types of foods in one meal or snack. Instead, try combining any foods in these separate groups with vegetables or salads. Experiment to find which foods and combinations work best for you.

### Milking Your Health

The old axiom is "cow's milk is for calves, human milk is for humans." Unfortunately, more people hear the "Got Milk?" ads than heed professional recommendations. Milk consumption is up, and so are the problems created by it. In many people, milk can cause various types of gastrointestinal stress, skin problems and lowered immunity to infections and allergies. And worse, bovine growth hormone used by some dairy farmers to increase milk production is associated with the growth of cancer cells, specifically breast cancer in women. For most people, however, the problems with milk are more subtle and affect quality of life.

The proteins in cow milk are more difficult for the human intestinal tract to digest and for the immune system to tolerate than are the proteins in human milk. Cow milk is about 80 percent casein and 20 percent whey while human milk is just the opposite, at 20 percent casein and 80 percent whey. A milk allergy is a true allergic reaction by the body's immune system to casein. Most of the time, symptoms are immediate and typically include swelling, itching, hives, abdominal cramping, breathing difficulty and diarrhea. Sometimes, chronic constipation is the result. In a severe reaction, hypotension or shock can result.

Lactose, or milk sugar, poses another potential problem with milk, as many people have difficulty digesting this sugar and some cannot digest it at all. Those who have difficulty digesting lactose do not produce enough of an enzyme called lactase, which breaks down the complex lactose into simple sugars. In these people, the lactose ferments in the small intestine, producing gas, bloating, cramps and diarrhea. Lactose-digestion problems are also associated with more serious problems such as irritable bowel syndrome, premenstrual syndrome and mental depression.

Many people who have problems with cow milk find that they can tolerate milk from sheep and goats much better. Sheep and goat milk are much closer in composition and overall nutrient content to human milk. Sheep milk can be difficult to obtain, but goat milk is widely available in many grocery stores. Like human milk, goat and sheep milk are higher in whey than casein. Goat milk is lower in lactose, and some say the lactose in sheep or goat milk is better tolerated by some people than lactose in cow milk. The fat in both goat and sheep milk is made up of smaller fat globules that are easier to digest.

## Say Cheese!

Cheeses made from the milk of cows, goats, sheep and other animals have been eaten by humans for thousands of years, and for many, cheese remains a good source of protein and other nutrients.

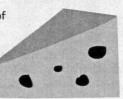

Making cheese basically involves removing liquid from the milk. This is normally achieved by heating the milk and adding a bacterial culture. The bacteria consume much of the lactose, producing lactic acid. This acid in turn causes the casein to form curd and separate from the whey. It is from this curd that most cheeses are made.

This is good news for those who are sensitive to lactose, because most of the milk sugar is either consumed by the bacteria or separates with the whey in the cheese-making process. For those who have problems digesting casein, though, many cheeses may not be well tolerated.

For those who are sensitive to casein, there are some types of cheeses made from whey. Ricotta, for example, is a soft cheese often, though not always, made from whey. With its whey protein and low lactose content, ricotta might be the best cheese choice for many people. And sheep or goat ricotta may be the best of the best. Many American-made ricottas are not made from whey, so read the labels. Italian and other specialty markets often have both soft and semi-soft ricottas.

## Wine, Alcohol and Your Health

Wine is not only the oldest alcoholic beverage but the oldest medicinal agent in continuous use throughout human history. The use of wine dates back more than 6,000 years, and is attributed to physicians, scientists, poets and peasants. Even today, wine and other alcoholic beverages are classified as foods and used daily in most cultures. More healthful benefits have been bestowed upon wine than any other natural substance. For instance, drinking wine with meals can help the digestive process.

There are few known unhealthy effects from moderate amounts of alcohol consumption, with negative consequences seen mostly in heavy drinkers. In fact, there are many positive health benefits associated with wine consumption. Drinking wine and other alcohol in moderation significantly lowers the risk of coronary heart disease. Moderate drinkers have healthier cholesterol ratios as alcohol raises the HDL and lowers LDL. This may be one reason for the lower incidence of heart disease in consumers versus abstainers. Another may be that alcohol increases blood flow to the heart. In addition, alcohol reduces the tendency to form blood clots, a major cause of heart attacks (and strokes). Alcohol also lowers the risk of Alzheimer's disease and other types of dementia. Moreover, those who don't drink actually have greater risk for heart disease. Some scientists say that people who have one or two drinks per day may add three to four years of life expectancy, as compared to those who don't drink.

Scientists also say that red wine may be a potent cancer inhibitor. Resveratrol, a substance found in red wine (due to the fact that grape skins are used to make red wine, but not white), grapes, peanuts, and thousands of medicinal plants from South America and China, not only interferes with cancer's development, but may also cause precancerous cells to reverse to normal. Resveratrol also has anti-inflammatory properties. (Other anti-inflammatory compounds, such as aspirin, are now associated with lower incidences of certain types of cancers due to their ability to inhibit tumor formation.)

Most wine contains about 12 percent alcohol (mostly ethanol, with only a very small percentage of other types of alcohol). Sweet dessert wines may contain up to 20 percent alcohol. This compares to 40 percent (80 proof) and 50 percent (100 proof) alcohol in distilled products such as vodka and gin. Wine also contains vitamins B1, B2, B6 and niacin, as well as traces of most minerals, including iron. Most red table wine contains iron in the easily usable ferrous form. The pH of wine is low, like that of the stomach, perhaps one reason wine improves appetite and digestion. Eating natural fats with wine slows the absorption of alcohol and protects the intestine from possible irritation.

Once in the blood, alcohol is destroyed in the liver. About 3.5 ounces of pure alcohol can be safely metabolized by the body if spread out over the day. This translates to about a bottle of wine — not something I'm recommending. To a European, this may not seem like excess, but to an American it might. In the United States, the average annual per capita consumption of wine is just a few teaspoons, while in Italy, it's about a half bottle.

As a group, women are more susceptible to negative effects of alcohol because of their smaller size, and the lesser amount of alcohol dehydrogenase in their stomachs. This enzyme breaks down much of the alcohol before it's absorbed.

If you enjoy wine and want the health benefits associated with it, drink only what you enjoy and can tolerate, and no more than one or two glasses. The simplest recommendation is a 4-ounce glass or two with meals. For most people a glass of wine will be completely metabolized in about an hour and a half. Some people, however, should never consume alcohol. But a moderate amount for those who can, and want to, is now considered to be 4 to 8 ounces of wine per day.

An obvious side effect of alcohol is that it impairs your senses, so it should be avoided within four hours of driving a vehicle. One drink increases the risk of an accident by 50 percent, two drinks by 100 percent. Also, wine should not be taken with other drugs, or by people with certain illnesses, and is not recommended for pregnant women. If you enjoy wine, be sure to ask your doctor whether it poses any health problems for you.

## Coffee, Tea and Caffeine

Many people use caffeine as a drug, as a means of getting more "energy." If this is the case with you, you may be addicted. And if you need a drug to give you a pick up, your energy-generating mechanism — the fat-burning aerobic system — is probably not working very well. Caffeine can also induce adrenal, liver and nervous-system stress, and create unstable blood-sugar levels in many people. As with everything else, you must determine whether your body can tolerate caffeine from coffee or tea. If you can, there are some important considerations.

Coffee beans are high in polyunsaturated oils, which can become rancid if left exposed to oxygen. The best way to avoid this oxidized oil is to buy your beans as freshly roasted as possible, keep them in the freezer, and grind them just before you make the coffee. Also, the darker the roast, the more the bean is roasted, and the more the oils are heated. Try to pick lighter roasts, which are heated less. But remember, the lighter roasts have more caffeine. Just as with fruits and vegetables, it's best to choose organic coffee to avoid chemical fertilizers, pesticides and other chemicals.

Many health benefits have been associated with both green and black tea, including anti-cancer properties, since they contain a variety of antioxidants and phytonutrients. Once again, organic tea is better than conventional as tea growers may use many pesticides.

If you can tolerate caffeine, two or three cups of coffee a day are usually the maximum for good health — you can drink more tea since it contains less caffeine. If you enjoy coffee but can't take the caffeine, whole-bean coffees that are water-processed to remove most of the caffeine are an alternative. But remember, not all the caffeine is eliminated in this coffee; as much as a third remains. So three cups of this decaf may equal one cup of regular. Decaf tea is also available, but if you want to avoid caffeine, use herbal teas such as peppermint or chamomile.

### Good News for Cocoa Lovers

The evidence is growing that cocoa is a powerful therapeutic food. Including this treat in the diet may do more than satisfy a craving — it may also help to improve health. Cocoa can help lower blood pressure and improve cardiovascular health. Researchers recently suggested that flavanols found in cocoa, purple grape juice and tea can stimulate processing of nitric oxide, which promotes healthy blood flow and blood pressure, and cardiovascular health. In addition, recent research confirms other studies indicating that flavanol-rich cocoa may work much like aspirin to promote healthy blood flow by preventing blood platelets from sticking together.

In addition to flavanols, cocoa contains other nutrients for good health. Depending on how it's processed, cocoa typically contains significant protein content of about 7 or 8 grams per ounce. It is also low in carbohydrate — between 8 and 13 grams per ounce, with 50 to 60 percent or more of that carbohydrate coming in the form of fiber. Like other beans, cocoa contains many vitamins and minerals, including folic acid, niacin, zinc and magnesium.

The fats in natural cocoa also have healthy attributes. More than a third of the fat in cocoa is oleic acid, the monounsaturated fat that gives olive oil its health benefits. An equal amount of fat in cocoa is in the form of stearic acid. Though saturated, stearic acid is a good fat, as it can reduce LDL cholesterol. Cocoa also contains the essential fat linoleic acid.

Cocoa also has strong antioxidant benefits, which have also been shown specifically to protect against LDL-cholesterol damage. One study showed that when a cocoa snack was substituted for a high-carbohydrate snack, it increased the "good" HDL cholesterol and reduced blood triglycerides. And, it did not increase LDL cholesterol despite being a higher-fat snack.

Polyphenols in cocoa, similar to those in red wine, provide protection against blood-vessel problems, including heart disease.

While cocoa has some very healthy attributes, eating it in a candy bar is not recommended since this usually includes a lot of sugar, bad fats and chemicals. Use cocoa in healthy products, or use it to make your own healthy desserts.

### Salt of the Sea

If you like salt and if you are not sodium sensitive, sea salt can be a flavorful and healthful addition to your food. Sea salt tastes like regular salt, but it has a better balance of minerals and also contains many trace minerals the body requires. Early humans obtained much of their food from the salt-water ocean, and we still require many of the sea's vital minerals.

People have come to fear sodium these days, almost as much as fats. However, like fat, sodium is an essential nutrient. It is needed by the body for water regulation, nervous-system and muscle activity, adrenal-gland function and many other essential actions.

Normal sodium intake through your daily diet is the best defense against sodium depletion, which can be a real problem especially in those who sweat or work out a lot. Read labels, because "low sodium" products abound on the market. Some people, due to adrenal stress, are often in need of more sodium because they lose a lot throughout the day (through the urine). Although they generally crave salt, a classic symptom, they are afraid to eat it. The unlimited use of sea salt is recommended for athletes, assuming they are not salt sensitive.

About one-third to one-half of those with hypertension are sodium sensitive; too much sodium may cause edema and/or an elevation of blood pressure. This sensitivity can be discovered through a good case history and examination by a health-care professional, and by avoiding all salt and sodium for a week and checking how blood pressure changes.

### Spice Up Your Health

Spices have been used in food preparation for thousands of years. The right spice, or combination of spices, can make foods tempting and delicious by boosting the appearance, smell and taste. Spices also are useful as natural preservatives, and have powerful therapeutic and health-promoting properties, too. In food, spices can prevent the growth of dangerous bacteria and other organisms. And when ingested, they can fight against cancer, heart disease and other chronic conditions. In most cases, it's the essential oils that are the protective and therapeutic components, partly due to their antioxidant and phytonutrient properties.

Oregano, thyme and bay leaf can protect against potentially harmful infectious agents such as Candida, E. coli, Salmonella and Staph, and even the potentially deadly Klebsiella pneumoniae.

Ginger, a common spice in oriental foods, is a highly effective anti-inflammatory agent, as are rosemary, turmeric (which contains the antioxidant curcumin) and capsaicin (from hot red pepper). The anti-inflammatory properties of these spices give them value as cancer preventatives. Ginger can also inhibit the rhinovirus — one of the viruses responsible for the common cold. Ginger's antioxidant properties are at least as effective as those of vitamin C. Ginger is also very useful for nausea and motion sickness, and can help protect the intestine from ulcers. In addition, ginger may have properties that promote fat burning.

Other hot spices also have beneficial properties. Capsaicin can stimulate increased oxygen uptake, which is one reason it may also increase fat-burning capability. Wasabi, a hot root used with Japanese foods, also protects against potential food poisoning by bacteria and fungus. It also contains anti-cancer properties, including powerful antioxidants.

Parsley not only adds a visual pleasure to a plate of food, but is also a seasoning that's full of phytonutrients, as well as the traditional minerals and vitamins with antioxidant effects. Fenugreek (the seed) contains high levels of flavanoids — an important antioxidant. Fenugreek has been shown to have cholesterol-lowering capabilities. This spice can also reduce platelet aggregation (important for proper blood flow), and can reduce blood sugar in diabetics.

Many other herbs and spices have therapeutic value as well, including cinnamon, allspice, nutmeg, cloves, dill, and basil. These can be found fresh in groceries or can be grown in your garden, window box or even an inside window sill. Dried spices can lose not only their flavor but also their therapeutic value over time, as many potent substances break down. And, since they contain polyunsaturated oils, they can go rancid. Buy spices in small packages, keep them sealed tightly and stored in a cool, dark place.

As you can see, there are many more aspects to your dietary health than merely balancing your macronutrients and micronutrients. By paying attention to some of these finer points of diet and nutrition you will become more intuitive about what is healthy and not healthy for your body. For those who need a little help getting started there are "diet" programs, which are discussed in the next chapter. And by all means, enjoy!

# 21 One Last Bite

Just as each of us has a different set of fingerprints, specific dietary requirements vary greatly from person to person. Therefore no one "diet" can work for all individuals. To build and maintain good function, you must supply your diet with the right mix of fuels and nutrients that are specific to your own individual needs. Rigid diets that specify what foods you should and shouldn't eat can't work for everyone. Some people thrive on a vegetarian diet; others need meat to be healthy. Some have allergies to different kinds of foods, and all of us have unique food preferences. Your job is to find out what works best for you. Throughout the previous chapters, you have been given the tools to help you do just that.

One of the most worrisome and disruptive developments that has taken place within the natural-health field has been the trend toward cookbook diet formulas. There are dozens of diet plans claiming to have the right answer for everyone. While diets such as these may work for some people, they can create dietary or nutritional imbalances for others.

In this chapter I briefly discuss a few important aspects of the diet not mentioned previously in this book. These include three common approaches to "dieting" used today: calorie-counting, which is still the most common approach; the infamous low-fat diet; and measuring grams of carbohydrates, fats and proteins, together with using percentages of macronutrients. Each one has some good and bad points associated with it, and they all have some common denominators. But the bottom line is that none of them will work for everyone. At best, they can act as a stepping stone for you, on your way to intuitively and instinctively knowing what is best for your body.

## Counting Calories

The calorie-counting theory is based on the idea that the calories in the food you eat, minus the calories you burn for energy, equals the weight you lose or gain. The idea is that balancing energy intake and output results in stable weight. If you eat fewer calories than you burn, you lose weight. But if you take in more than you use, you gain. The problem with this theory is that it does not work as simply as it seems for most people. The reason is that everyone has a different metabolism, so food is utilized differently, and fat and sugar are burned at different ratios from person to person. For example, some people get 60 percent of energy from fat and 40 percent from sugar, while others are just the opposite.

In addition to the number of calories taken in, the amount of carbohydrates, fats and proteins eaten also significantly affects how the body burns energy. So to use only the total calories as a guide may be misleading. In addition, calorie counting does not consider where those calories come from, the quality of food, or the balance of macronutrients. More importantly, counting calories doesn't work in real life and the side effects can be significant — the least damaging being weight gain as a result of slowing down your metabolism.

### Case History

*When Sally turned 30, she decided to get serious about taking off the excess weight. So she followed a low-calorie diet that limited her intake to 1,000 calories per day. Within three months, Sally felt more tired, but finally reached her goal of losing 20 pounds. Within six months, she gained about 25 pounds back. She went back on her diet, and it was just as successful as before, although it took a little longer to lose the 25 pounds. This vicious cycle continued for about five years. Sally was now not only tired, but depressed, had insomnia, and had PMS for two weeks each month. During my initial consultation with Sally, I explained how she was continually suppressing her metabolism and getting more unhealthy with each vicious cycle. Sally was weaned off her calorie counting and eventually was able to eat as much as her body required. In time she got down to the same size clothes she wore when she was at her "ideal" weight at 22 years of age. And to her surprise, she was eating about 2,000 calories each day!*

Calorie counting almost always results in eating less food. When you eat less food, especially less fat, which contains the most calories, one of the significant results can be that your metabolism slows down and you can eventually store more fat, despite your initial (short-term) weight loss. That's why so many people eventually gain more weight and fat after being on a calorie-restricted diet. The best way to speed up metabolism is to eat the amount of good-quality food you need each day. Other factors that increase the metabolism are dietary fats and aerobic exercise.

### Low-Fat Diets

One of the most popular and health-damaging diet plans is the low-fat diet. The basic idea is built on the fallacy that dietary fat only causes weight gain and is detrimental to health. Some people on low-fat diets avoid fat like the plague and often develop "fat-phobia." Low-fat diets are also popular among calorie-counters because they are a seemingly easy way to reduce calories.

There are several problems associated with low-fat diets, many of which are the same as those associated with low-calorie diets. Low-fat diets can slow metabolism, and also increase hunger through reduced satiety. People on low-fat diets also tend to eat more carbohydrate; as you may recall, 40 percent or more of carbohydrate is directly converted to fat for storage by the body.

But the worst problems associated with low-fat diets are essential-fatty-acid imbalances, hormonal problems and disease. Essential fatty acids are usually deficient in low-fat diets, along with all the benefits previously explained in chapters 9 and 11. Women who are on or who have been on low-fat diets are especially vulnerable to hormonal imbalances. And finally, contrary to popular belief, low-fat diets do not prevent disease. In fact, some types of fat are associated with prevention of heart disease and cancer, as discussed in previous chapters.

**The Gram Counter**
Knowing the weight in grams of each food eaten at a meal can have more practical meaning than knowing the calories of that meal. Counting grams at least considers all the macronutrients individually. The best example is determining how many grams of carbohydrate there are in a given food or meal, and the ratio of carbohydrate to protein. Along with other factors, this measurement has an important relationship with the amount of insulin produced by the pancreas. For example, a good starting point is to have about a 2:1 ratio of carbohydrate to protein. For some this works very well, but others may need even more protein and less carbohydrate.

Gram counting also includes the popular 40-30-30 plan, which suggests people eat 40 percent of their calories from carbohydrates, and 30 percent each from protein and fat. Note that this refers to percentages of calories, not percentages of grams. Calculating the percentages requires some math skill. You must multiply the grams of each macronutrient by 4 calories for carbohydrate, 4 for protein, and 9 for fat, and divide each subtotal by the total calories of the food or meal. (Fats have 9 calories per gram, and carbohydrates and proteins each have 4 calories per gram.)

But counting grams, like counting calories, can also maintain the dieting obsession. Each time you eat something you have to think about how much it weighs or you have to look it up in a food table. Most people eventually get tired of doing that and fall off their "diet."

### Follow Your Intuition

If all this sounds too complicated, you're right. Why count calories or grams? Why blindly follow some menu when you can do what every other animal on earth does — eat when you're hungry, eat what you feel your body needs, and stop when you're satisfied?

Unfortunately, none of the popular diet approaches consider how you respond to your meals. Do they make you feel more hungry? Tired? Energized? How you feel immediately after a meal, and for the next few hours, is one of the best indicators of whether that type of meal works well for your needs. As you consider this and other factors we've discussed in previous chapters, you'll be on your way to knowing what works best for you. What is really happening, is you're developing your natural intuition.

For many people a plan that makes sense is to determine the types and amounts of foods that work best for you, and then devise a schedule that divides this food up over the course of the day. Typically this means three regular meals with two or three healthy snacks as discussed in chapter 19. Eating right is often a matter of planning. You plan your day, often writing it down in your planner; you plan the clothes you're going to wear and you plan vacations. If you plan your meals as carefully, you'll be much healthier. Let's plan a day's menu, beginning with the breaking of your all-night fast, breakfast.

### Breakfast

There's no better way to start your day than with a healthy breakfast. For many people, this includes some quality protein. Keeping your carbohydrate foods to the proper level will help optimize blood sugar, which will give you more physical and mental energy for the day's tasks ahead. On the other hand, cereal, doughnuts or pancakes will get your day off to a bad start.

Eggs are the perfect breakfast food. While they're not just for breakfast, they just could make your first meal of the day ideal, and a bit easier to prepare — whether poached, scrambled, soft-boiled, fried, hard-boiled or in an omelet.

Omelets are great because they can include a serving or two of vegetables, and also provide a change of pace. On weekends, when you have more time to prepare breakfast, a fancy omelet with a sauce makes for a nice change. Another version of the omelet is quiche, made with vegetables, meat or fish. You'll want to make this ahead of time to reduce cooking time in the morning.

Eggs can also be added to a fruit smoothie in the blender. In this case, avoid the raw whites because they contain an enzyme, avidin, which may interfere with your body's ability to make and use the nutrient biotin. The yolk does not contain avidin. Smoothies can also be made from plain yogurt (avoid the sweet types), one egg yolk (or more), and fresh fruit. If you find some blueberries or strawberries that you just love, buy a lot of them and store them in the freezer. To make your smoothie, just throw them in frozen. Many people like peanut or almond butter or use whole nuts or seeds in their smoothies. Don't be afraid to experiment.

Don't have time for breakfast? Make time. There are several things you can do to ensure you get this most important first meal of the day. First, do as much preparation as possible the night before. Not just breakfast prep, but things you do in the morning, like pack your briefcase, set out your clothes or pack your bags. As for meal preparation, get everything out and ready to go, except for the food itself; put water in the kettle, pan on the stove, plate, silverware and napkin on the table.

Egg breakfasts can be your staple, and with so many varieties there's no need to be bored with them. But maybe you still want more variety or are really in a hurry, so here's another healthy breakfast variation: cottage cheese, or real ricotta cheese. Combine it with anything you want that doesn't contain refined sugar and you've got a really quick, easy and healthy meal. Cottage or ricotta cheese with fresh fruit makes a really quick breakfast. Look for cheese with the least amount of ingredients, especially those with names you can't pronounce. Some people like these cheeses as part of a smoothie.

Whatever you choose to have for breakfast, just remember it's the most important meal of the day, so don't cheat yourself or your family out of it.

## Lunch

If you eat a good breakfast, and a mid-morning snack, getting to lunch without crawling on your knees from hunger should not be a problem. And like breakfast, a healthy lunch is a matter of proper planning. Packing your own lunch usually makes for a more healthful midday meal. If you are bringing your lunch to work or school, you can arrange for that to be done the evening before so it's not another job you need to do in the morning. Plan ahead by cooking extra food at dinner so that you have leftovers for lunch.

Eating more protein and less carbohydrate during lunch will keep you from getting sleepy or losing concentration after lunch. So choose the meat or fish and vegetable, rather than the pasta, potato and bread. And avoid dessert.

Leftovers from a balanced dinner make for a perfect lunch — perhaps a few slices of beef or a chunk of fish with steamed vegetables and a small side of rice. While the traditional sandwich often comes to mind at lunchtime, for those who are carbohydrate intolerant or who have problems with wheat, how about serving some tuna, chicken or ham salad, along with some sliced avocado on top of a salad for lunch? Use a plastic or glass container, fill it with vegetables such as leaf lettuce, carrots, avocado, red peppers, celery, tomatoes, etc., and top it off with the tuna, chicken, eggs or ham salad, or any meat, fish or cheese. If you're making a salad out of tuna, chicken or whatever, be sure to use only a mayonnaise that has healthy oil in it. An olive oil or canola-oil mayo is the best, and contains a lot of monounsaturated oil.

If you're going out for lunch, make sure you take enough time so you're not rushed. And if you have the habit of grabbing some food and eating at your desk, break it. You'll be much more productive taking the break. Don't be afraid to have eggs again as an option; they're a quick meal you can get almost anywhere. Just beware of the greasy grills.

No time for lunch? If you work for a company, there are laws about taking adequate lunch periods. If you work for yourself, make your own rules. Of course, you first have to be convinced that your meals are a priority. Even a 30-minute lunch period is enough time to eat a relaxed and healthy meal.

## Dinner

If you start the day with a real breakfast, have a good lunch, and eat healthy snacks, dinner should be your smallest meal. This is the ideal scenario. Too often, however, people do just the opposite. They skip breakfast, have a skimpy lunch and then pile on the food in the evening. My dinner at home is typically an appetizer-size plate of something, like a small Romaine salad with shrimp, or a small serving of beef and steamed vegetables with a wine sauce, and a glass of wine, or even some avocado dip with vegetables. Your dinner could include items from the refrigerator that you combine for a sampling of leftovers you've accumulated over the past few days. Or, once again, eggs can be a great dinner. Or it could be just a small salad. Either way, dinner should be easy, relaxing and small.

## Sauces Make Food Taste Better

Whether it's breakfast, lunch or dinner, any meal can be made more savory and even romantic with a sauce. When you think of a sauce, the thought of preparation time first comes to mind. But some basic sauce recipes are quick, easy and store well. They can turn your seemingly simple and boring meals into culinary delights. Below are three basic sauce recipes that you can make with very little preparation time, and the results will keep well for use a second or third time. You may also find yourself feasting on just the sauce!

A note about recipes: I learned to cook by intuition, "throwing ingredients into the pot" rather than by following a recipe and measuring everything. I recommend you do the same. Over time, you'll make more delicious meals in less time and without the anxiety often associated with following a recipe. I do, however, highly recommend reading through cookbooks to get more ideas about combining ingredients.

## Basic Butter Sauce

The most basic of sauces is also the easiest to make — a butter sauce. When you make your vegetables, put some "sweet" butter on the vegetables when they're still hot, along with some sea salt. ("Sweet" butter is made without salt — the cream used to make this butter is a higher quality and more tasty than that used for salted butter.) Even those who never liked vegetables will usually eat them with a butter sauce. Don't be afraid to use generous amounts of both ingredients, unless there's a real reason to limit these ingredients in your diet. This is the real key to a great butter sauce. If you have the time and want to get more fancy, sauté some garlic or onions, with or without some spices (tarragon works well), in butter, with some olive oil. Add salt and you have a variation of the basic butter sauce. Prep time is just 20 seconds for the basic sauce, and less than 5 minutes for the fancy butter sauce with garlic.

## Basic Tomato Sauce

This is a quick and easy, tasty and healthy all-around red sauce. Just put some chopped tomatoes with a small amount of water in an uncovered pot, add some sea salt and let it simmer for a couple of hours, or more if you want a thicker, tastier sauce and you have time. If you can't get fresh, vine-ripened tomatoes, use canned, whole, peeled organic tomatoes which are vine ripened and packed without preservatives. The canned ones are easier and quicker to make. When cooked down to a thicker puree, tomatoes take on a unique taste all their own and even without adding anything but salt, you'll have a great-tasting sauce. If you like tomato sauce, you'll love this simple way of making it. It's a guarantee that people who taste it will ask for the recipe! You can freeze this sauce in small containers and use it when you want. Once you have the basic sauce, if time permits, you can add other ingredients, like garlic, parsley, or your grandmother's favorite spices. But a sprinkle of Parmesan or Romano cheese is all you'll need. Also, try adding a scoop of sour cream or ricotta cheese to this basic tomato sauce.

### Basic Cream Sauce

The fanciest of basic sauces is the cream sauce. This is simply made from heavy cream, butter, flour and salt. Use the same amount of cream as the amount of sauce you want. For example, for about 2 cups of sauce, use a bit less than 2 cups of cream. Heat the cream to just before it simmers. In a separate pan, melt about a half stick of unsalted butter on low heat. With a whisk, slowly stir in about three tablespoons of whole-wheat flour into the butter (pastry flour works best). Slowly add the hot cream while continually stirring over low to medium heat, bringing to a simmer for five to 10 minutes. Add sea salt to taste.

Once you can make a good basic cream sauce quickly and easily, you can make a variety of different, more fancy sauces almost as easily. For example, adding some chopped onion or garlic, bay leaf or other ingredients to the cream, after heating it, makes a different sauce. For a cheese sauce, add some grated Parmesan or Romano cheese. For a wine sauce, add a couple of tablespoons of red wine or sherry.

### Eating on the Run

The realities of life dictate that you won't always be able to eat the way that's best. When you travel, are late for work, or somehow find you can't get a good meal when you need it, you'll have to find the best alternative. There are some acceptable options. If you're away from home and are having trouble finding good food, consider going to a deli for a chef's salad, or just some sliced meats and cheeses. If you can tolerate bread, a deli sandwich made with whole-wheat bread is better than fried or fast foods. Another option is to go to a diner. Here you can always get eggs cooked sunny-side up or poached to avoid too much grease. Pass on the omelets or scrambled eggs during busy hours when they often make these dishes from a big pot of eggs broken far ahead of time. In some restaurants, prepackaged liquid eggs are used for scrambled eggs and omelets. Also be sure to ask if they use margarine. If they don't have real butter, have your toast dry. Cottage cheese and fresh fruit is also easy to get at a diner.

Another alternative is to eat a healthy energy bar. Unfortunately, you'll have a difficult time finding one that is acceptable. You can buy some ahead of time and always have some on hand at home and work. Read labels and buy bars made only from real-food ingredients. Avoid energy bars that contain corn syrup, hydrogenated or fractionated oils and synthetic vitamins. Most so-called energy bars on the market are full of artificial or processed foods and/or vitamins, and are not recommended. The same is true for snack drinks; use only the ones made from good ingredients. I've formulated my own real-food bars and drinks; Phil's

Bars™, Alma bars™ and Phil's Shakes™ are made from all real food with no hydrogenated fat, MSG or synthetic vitamins.

Whether you're eating a meal or a snack, choose food that's in the most natural state possible. And, eating a variety of foods, in the form of vegetables, fruits, meats and fish, will help you get your full spectrum of nutrients from natural sources.

## Foods for Children

One of the most common dietary questions I receive from people relates to feeding their children. The answer, in principle, is relatively simple. From baby's first foods, they eat the same things adults eat, sometimes in a different form. The implementation is not always so easy, mostly due to marketing of junk foods to children. Let's start at the beginning.

From birth, mother's milk provides everything the baby needs, including water. It's not unusual for a baby to rely exclusively on breastfeeding for all its nutritional needs through 6 or 8 months of age, or longer. I've never seen a situation where the mother was physically unable to breastfeed. If you're expecting a baby and would like more information and support on breastfeeding, contact La Leche League International (1-800-La Leche).

The general recommendation is to wait until at least 6 to 8 months of age before introducing outside sources of food for babies (although baby food companies want you to think differently). A baby's intestinal tract is not yet developed to process food other than mother's milk, and the immune system could have adverse reactions to foreign foods if they're introduced too early. This could lead to intestinal problems, allergies and other problems, often for a lifetime. When babies start wanting to experiment with food after 6 to 8 months of age, you can begin trying different foods individually. If you combine more than one food at a time in the beginning and the baby has an adverse reaction, you may not know which food is the culprit. And, it's best to give the baby a choice, letting him or her choose from a variety of healthy options.

Babies are born as instinctive and intuitive geniuses; they know just what they need to be healthy. And when they start eating foods, they can self-select very well, when not influenced by adults or other kids. Studies by Dr. Clara Davis in the 1920s and '30s showed that once children are weaned, they will naturally select the foods their bodies need the most. In Davis' studies, the children developed very different dietary patterns. In the end, the children were psychologically and physically healthier than average.

Practically speaking, most parents are not willing to prepare a smorgasbord for the baby every time he or she wants to eat. But there are some patterns I discuss below that can be followed — mainly that certain foods, like carbohydrates and dairy products, should be postponed until they are more easily tolerated, and more-often selected foods should be eaten first.

The best first foods to introduce are vegetables. Letting the baby play with a fresh raw carrot, zucchini or other raw vegetables (except potatoes since even a small amount of hidden sprout can be toxic) can be a great way to introduce food. Use larger vegetables, or pieces, so the baby can't get it stuck in the mouth. Regardless, you'll want to keep close — infants seem to get any size item into their mouths one way or another. Eventually they'll figure out they can get pieces of the vegetables with their new teeth. Try one vegetable at a time and see which they like, which, if any, they react badly to, and if they really have an interest. Some babies just want to play with food, just as with everything else around them. If they don't seem ready to eat, don't push it. Wait a couple of weeks and introduce some raw vegetables again.

Next move on to cooked vegetables — peas, squash, carrots or whatever you're eating. Just mash up the vegetables you cook for yourself and feed them to the baby. Hold the butter and salt until a couple of months later. Also keep away from rough or hard-to-digest vegetables like artichokes and those in the cabbage family, including broccoli, cauliflower and Brussels sprouts. You'll gradually see what your baby likes, and what his or her system can handle, when you change diapers.

Once a variety of vegetables is tolerated, start next with fruits. Try a large piece of apple, pear or peach. Don't forget, the baby's goal is to get it into his or her mouth — whole, of course. Move on to applesauce, and try pear and peach sauce too, preferably all homemade. Avoid using fruit juice; it's too concentrated, and even if you dilute it you'll increase acidity in the baby's mouth which will have a devastating effect on the teeth, leading to tooth decay later.

Now that the baby is eating fresh vegetables and fruits, you're ready to experiment with cooked eggs (initially try the yolk and white separately in case there's a reaction to either), meats and fish. Buy everything as fresh as possible, avoiding the processed meats and canned foods, and choosing certified organic whenever possible. Make dairy and grains the very last foods you introduce. Milk and wheat are the most common allergies in children, followed by soy and corn. Why not hold off on these potential problems as long as possible since the baby will get everything he or she needs nutritionally from the other foods?

So much of the food preferences people develop later in life were acquired at an early age from what their parents fed them as babies. Starting off right makes feeding your older, more picky children much easier. The bottom line is this: If your kids are not eating right it's usually your fault. In their early years, take the responsibility to buy and prepare all the food they eat. Don't let the processed-food companies and the lure of convenience dictate how your child will eat for the rest of his or her life. The quality of your child's entire life depends on it.

# EXERCISING YOUR OPTIONS

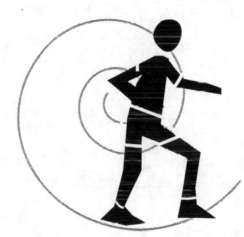

# 22 Developing Maximum Aerobic Function

Earlier in this book we defined fitness as a crucial element to human perform-ance. In the purest sense, fitness is the ability to perform physical activity. For most of their existence humans were extremely active, expending vast amounts of energy just to accomplish the basic tasks that kept them alive, like walking for miles in search of food. These early people had tremendous endurance based on aerobic systems that were built by their daily tasks of living. In just a short peri-od of a couple of generations, today's humans have become much less active and as a consequence we are much more prone to dysfunction and disease. Most peo-ple don't get enough aerobic exercise, and many who do exercise get too much anaerobic work, which can be very stressful, causing injury and illness.

All through this book I've also discussed the concept of getting more energy from fat. It's no coincidence that the aerobic system uses mostly fat as fuel, while the anaerobic system uses mostly sugar. It follows that to improve your level of fitness, enhance your ability to burn fat, obtain unlimited energy and correct most bodily imbalances, the aerobic system must be revved up. It's up to you to develop as much aerobic function as possible. I refer to this as *Maximum Aerobic Function*, or MAF.

You actually have two very different types of cells in your muscles, com-prising aerobic and anaerobic fibers. In some animals, such as chickens, the aero-bic and anaerobic muscle fibers are separate, with entire muscles composed of one or the other. When cooked, a chicken clearly shows this distinction — dark meat is composed of aerobic muscle fibers, while white meat is anaerobic muscle.

In humans, all muscles have a mixture of both aerobic and anaerobic fibers. The aerobic muscle fibers make up the foundation of the aerobic system. These fibers account for the majority of muscle bulk in the human body, more than 80 percent of all the fibers. This fact corresponds to the ability of humans to be better endurance animals than sprinters.

Aerobic muscle fibers have two general functions: physical activity including support, and metabolic function. Aerobic muscle fibers physically get us through the day and they're the ones we want working during physical perform-ance. They allow us to sit, type and walk throughout the day. These fibers, much more than the anaerobic ones, provide protection for the spine, hips and all other joints and bones. Without good aerobic muscle function, we're more vulnerable to stress fractures, joint problems and weakened bones.

**169**

Your aerobic muscles must be physically active for the aerobic system to function well and for you to be healthy. Since most people are no longer naturally active, artificial activity, otherwise known as exercise, is necessary. The amount and intensity of your exercise is a key factor, which I'll discuss in detail in later chapters. Briefly, aerobic muscles are relatively slow-action muscles, capable of enduring easy to moderate levels of activity for long periods of time. This means you should be able to endure a long day's work without getting exhausted, and still have energy to play.

The aerobic fibers are well endowed with blood vessels, so the more these muscles are used, the more blood flows through them and the entire body. This improvement in circulation brings more oxygen to all cells, and removes waste products, which are always being produced. Conversely, the person who is very inactive may have 70 percent of his or her blood vessels closed down!

The metabolic aspect of aerobic muscle fiber is the other key component of the aerobic system. Within these fibers we produce long-term energy, specifically by converting fat to energy in the part of the muscle cells called the mitochondria. These fat-burning engines have iron-containing myoglobin, and require many other nutrients. As fat-burning improves, your body gets an unlimited supply of energy, and the fat deposits on your hips, thighs, abdomen and even in your arteries will diminish.

The aerobic fiber's numerous mitochondria also help antioxidants break down potentially dangerous free radicals. Taking all the antioxidants you need won't help if your aerobic system is not working efficiently.

In addition to aerobic and anaerobic muscle fibers, there is a third type, a mixed variety. These "mixed fibers" are best defined as aerobic, with potential anaerobic characteristics. Actually, you decide how these fibers are "programmed" — as aerobic, fat-burning fibers generating long-term energy, or as anaerobic sugar-burners that have limited energy potential. The mixed fibers are highly influenced by diet and exercise.

### Rescuing Your Aerobic System

To get your aerobic system working correctly, you must diminish or avoid factors that suppress it, and increase the factors that help it. I will briefly describe them here. More detailed discussions are contained in the coming chapters.

The biggest negative factor to your aerobic system is stress. The different types of stress and how to control them are discussed later in this book. For now it's important just to know that stress of any kind programs your body to burn less fat and more sugar. The more stress, the worse this problem will be.

Dietary or nutritional factors that cause excess stress can especially inhibit aerobic function. The most common of these stresses is eating too much refined carbohydrate foods and products containing sugar. Deficiencies of essential fats or other nutrients can also inhibit aerobic progress.

The other major lifestyle stress that suppresses the aerobic system is physical. This is often due to overexercising, and most commonly from too much anaerobic exercise. This important issue is discussed in the next chapter.

If the aerobic system is suppressed, energy needs switch from fat-burning toward using more sugar. This results in a deficiency in aerobic function, resulting in a variety of signs and symptoms I call Aerobic Deficiency Syndrome.

## Aerobic Deficiency Syndrome

*Aerobic Deficiency Syndrome* (ADS) is not an epidemic so easily defined that it makes big news each day, like Acquired Immune Deficiency Syndrome or heart disease. But this problem is destroying the quality of life for millions of people. It's one of the major causes of functional illness, and too often, the long-term result of ADS is major disease such as heart disease, cancer or diabetes.

This deficiency occurs when the aerobic system is not well developed and maintained. It's no different from vitamin C deficiency, or being deprived of any other necessity of life. It can cause problems in any area of the body dependent upon the aerobic system. If your risk for heart disease is high, for example, that may be the area most affected. If you have a family history of diabetes, aerobic deficiency can further increase your risk. Others may suffer a knee injury, back pain, exhaustion or some other less-threatening symptoms. A primary aerobic deficiency can cause many different end results in the form of secondary symptoms. These often become the target of therapies, with the primary problem, ADS, neglected. In general, the two most common causes of ADS are:

•The underuse of aerobic muscles. It's true, you must "use it or lose it." Only a small percentage of the population is either naturally active (their day-to-day work activity is high, as with construction workers, loggers, etc.) or performs aerobic exercise regularly (that which is easy, slow, and endurance-oriented). Of those who do exercise, too few do so in a way that really improves the aerobic system sufficiently. Some who are active, like those who walk to the office from the train station in New York City, may be too stressed to benefit from that activity.

• The overuse of anaerobic muscles. Most exercisers overtrain by performing too much anaerobic activity, such as weight-lifting, or activities performed at too high an intensity.

Other common causes of ADS include consumption of too much carbohydrate, including sugars; low-fat diets; and many lifestyle factors that suppress adrenal-gland function.

When asking yourself about the status of your aerobic system, do an inventory of all the functions with which the aerobic system is associated. The symptoms of ADS are many; the most common ones include:

• **Fatigue.** This is usually physical, but often can be mental. If you've ever visited a doctor with complaints of fatigue, he or she probably did a physical exam and then a blood test to rule out anemia or other clinical conditions. The doctor might have diagnosed your problem as chronic fatigue syndrome (which means you've been tired for a long time), but couldn't tell you what was causing it. Or maybe you were given the name of the latest virus. Worse yet, perhaps your doctor said you were getting old and fatigue is normal!

• **Recurrent injuries.** Do you know many people who don't have any type of injury? Shoulder and back pain, knee and wrist problems, weak ankles. It's not normal to have any injury at any age, even for people who exercise. When you have an injury, it means something went wrong and the end result is dysfunction in a joint, muscle, ligament or tendon. Most injuries are avoidable if proper balance is maintained in the body. If you have a properly functioning aerobic system, normal wear and tear on your body will be self-remedied because the aerobic muscle fibers are the main support for your joints and bones.

• **Excess storage of fat.** When the aerobic system doesn't work effectively, the body stores more fat. This fat can accumulate on the hips, thighs and abdomen, or in the arteries.

• **Blood-sugar stress.** It's abnormal to be hungry all the time. Cravings for sweets or stimulants like caffeine, tiredness after meals, moodiness, shakiness if you don't eat on time, or any symptom that comes on before you eat (and is relieved by eating) is often the result of blood-sugar instability.

- **Hormonal imbalance.** Premenstrual syndrome and menopausal symptoms are common in women with aerobic deficiency. This is partly due to a hormonal-system dysfunction, which depends on efficient aerobic activity and fat metabolism.

- **Circulatory problems.** Since so many of the body's blood vessels are found in the aerobic muscle fibers, a lack of aerobic function results in fewer operating blood vessels and diminished blood flow.

## Lactic Acid

Overuse of the anaerobic system can create a problem for the aerobic system due to the production of excess lactic acid. Problems occur when too much lactic acid is present in the body — either from too much anaerobic exercise or too little removal due to ADS. One clear result of too much lactic acid is further inhibition of the aerobic system.

Excess lactic-acid levels can also cause depression, anxiety, phobias and suicidal tendencies. It's even been shown that raising lactic-acid levels in normal, healthy people can produce these symptoms. This is probably due to the effect of lactic acid on the nervous system. Excess lactic acid can also disturb coordination. It's a cause for concern, especially in athletes and others who require a more finely tuned, coordinated body for their work or sport. A high-carbohydrate diet, too much refined-sugar intake and a low-fat diet can also aggravate high lactic-acid levels, as can various nutritional imbalances such as an increased need for thiamin.

Other symptoms related to higher lactic-acid levels include angina pectoris, seen in patients with certain heart problems. The heart is a muscle, and it's not immune to the damaging effects of lactic acid. High levels of lactic acid create a major stress on the heart and blood vessels and may aggravate existing problems such as high blood pressure and heart disease. This may be one reason why the incidence of heart attacks in people who are running or jogging is relatively high — a combination of ADS and excess lactic acid. It should be noted that anaerobic muscles normally produce lactic acid, and when entering the bloodstream lactic acid is converted to lactate.

## Aerobic Sex

One important and enjoyable function of human performance is the act of making love. Good aerobic capacity is an important ingredient for a good sex life. But for millions of people, poor sexual ability is a major stress.

There are many reasons for sexual dysfunction. While some sexual problems may be purely psychological, I don't feel qualified to help people with those kinds of imbalances. But I will say that when you are feeling generally fit and healthy, your psychological outlook often improves, too. And that includes a healthy interest in sex. That aside, it's the physiologic aspect I want to address, specifically, how a healthy aerobic system and adrenal sex hormones play a role in healthy sexual function. Even those without sexual problems may find they can improve an existing relationship by improving aerobic function.

If we look at the act of making love as a workout, we see a truer picture of what is happening. If one partner is always too tired in the evening, the problem often is aerobic deficiency. This may be caused by eating too many sweets or carbohydrate snacks in the course of the evening, or too much carbohydrate all day, especially in those who are carbohydrate intolerant.

Suppose the unresponsive partner isn't really tired. Perhaps that's the excuse used because he or she isn't especially aroused sexually. It may be a psychological problem, but for many, it isn't. This aspect of lovemaking is, for the most part, hormonal in nature, and sex hormones are affected by stress. Estrogen, for example, plays important roles, from arousal to lubrication. Testosterone also plays a vital role in sexual desire. Excess stress, a low-fat diet or other factors can reduce these hormones and have a devastating effect.

It is no coincidence that complaints of a lack of interest in sex often coincide with high stress states. In many people, this "sexual deficiency" then contributes even more to the already high stress level, and prevents the person from getting a much-needed stress reduction. Sexual activity can be very therapeutic. In the course of your day and week, all kinds of stress can accumulate. That tension, the increased sympathetic activity often associated with stress, if not balanced, can be harmful. The act of making love, specifically, having an orgasm, can eliminate that tension.

What of the complaint, often heard from women, that "he never lasts long enough?" Among the factors associated with this occurrence is a lack of stamina. This translates to endurance, or the lack of it. The inability to endure sexually is another symptom of aerobic deficiency. Correcting aerobic deficiency often eliminates these complaints.

Another factor associated with the person who "doesn't last long enough" is that he is usually not sufficiently warmed up. Many people, more often men, choose to make lovemaking a sprint rather than an endurance activity. In a later chapter I explain how a slow build-up of activity is vital to any workout. In this instance, the warm-up is very important, and can be accomplished with foreplay. Spending enough time warming up will allow the hormonal system to properly evoke the normal, healthy response in both partners. Without a warm-up, you may not be ready to continue effective, enjoyable sexual activity.

Cooling down is another aspect of sex too often neglected, just as in exercise; it's vital to the complete workout. Like warming up, or foreplay, cooling down is essential and should include a slow winding down, with easy, light-touch activity that produces even more feelings of relaxation. Using exercise as a pattern, making love requires the same elements: a slow increase in activity, followed by the peak of the workout, and ending with a cool-down.

There are a variety of dietary and nutritional factors that can help sexual performance. No, there's no pill that's a cookbook remedy despite all the ads for such gimmicks. The factors that really work happen to be the same ones that help improve overall aerobic and adrenal function as discussed in past chapters and in chapter 30. More importantly, there are a number of factors that can have a negative impact on sexual performance. These are, of course, the same factors that can inhibit aerobic function.

One aspect of sexual performance worth mentioning here is that of fertility. This problem can affect both males and females as potential parents. Women who want to conceive but are unable often suffer from a tremendous amount of stress. As natural as this may be, it doesn't make the process any easier, since stress further weakens the adrenal system, adversely affecting the hormones necessary to conceive.

The first step for a woman who cannot conceive (after several months of trying) is to be sure that ovulation is taking place, and that intercourse is taking place at the same time as ovulation. This can be done using a kit available from drug stores. If that doesn't result in success, make sure both partners have been examined and all physical or chemical reasons have been eliminated. If there are clear problems, your doctor will most likely have some recommended therapy. If no clear problems exist, you may be on your own again, unless you are willing to undergo more extreme hormonal therapy. This type of therapy never made sense to me for two reasons: It's not very successful; and it's relatively easy to improve aerobic function, which balances the hormonal status, often resulting in conception. If the more conservative approach fails, one still has the option to try more extreme measures.

The most common cause of infertility I have seen is carbohydrate intolerance, as described in chapter 6. Carbohydrate intolerance probably causes infertility by inhibiting some of the sex hormones (estrogen and progesterone). Alleviating carbohydrate intolerance through dietary changes also removes stress from the adrenal glands, which often increases DHEA and the sex hormones. Ultimately, this improves fertility, sometimes even in the most stubborn cases. (And sometimes when conception isn't wanted.)

In the case where fertility takes place but maintaining pregnancy is difficult, similar problems may exist. The difference is in the hormones that are most deficient. In many cases of early miscarriage, progesterone is too low. The same dietary factors may be important, but in addition, a natural preparation of progesterone may also be needed. Natural hormone therapy is discussed later, in chapter 30.

Sexual function is a normal, natural and healthy aspect of human performance, one that should take place throughout life, not just during youth. Imbalances in the aerobic system or the adrenal glands can adversely affect the sex hormones, resulting in sexual problems. Many common side effects of aerobic or stress-related dysfunction, such as fatigue, poor circulation or depression, can adversely affect sexual performance as well.

# 23 The Anaerobic Epidemic

Anaerobic muscle fibers allow us the power and speed we sometimes need in the course of the day. When we see great athletes on TV or in ads, it's often their anaerobic qualities that we find so impressive — speed, power and big muscles. The problem is that many people seek out this type of body at the expense of their aerobic systems, and therefore their health.

In order to be both fit and healthy, anaerobic function must be balanced with aerobic function. Unfortunately, most in our society are willing to improve their anaerobic systems even at the risk of losing aerobic function. Muscle machines, gyms with mirrors, and promises of "abs of steel" have attracted many exercisers. Bulking up has become analogous with health. However, adopting this philosophy can result in functional illness, and sometimes end in disease. Worse yet, we are educating our children to follow the same path by promoting no-pain, no-gain philosophies.

The anaerobic system includes the anaerobic muscle fibers, along with the related mechanisms used during high-stress activity. This system is associated with increased sugar-burning states, production of adrenal-stress hormones and the sympathetic nervous system. We couldn't survive without this mechanism, but when it's used too much, imbalances develop.

The imbalances caused by excess anaerobic function, physically developed through anaerobic exercise, can result frequently in injuries, illness, metabolic and hormonal imbalances, and added stress on the nervous system.

Metabolically speaking, the anaerobic system provides short-term energy, with these muscle fibers burning sugar, rather than fat, as an energy source. I emphasize again that it's important to burn sugar; we need it to maintain fat-burning, for brain energy, and as an additional source of physical energy, especially during stress. But it's a question of balance; too much anaerobic function results in an aerobic/anaerobic imbalance.

Imbalance can occur in someone with poor aerobic function, such as the out-of-shape person who relies on anaerobic energy because his aerobic system doesn't work well, or in an overtrained athlete who performs too much anaerobic work and too little aerobic exercise. The end result is they both develop the same type of imbalance with similar symptoms.

Excess anaerobic activity, whether by exercise, work stress, or diet, inhibits the aerobic system through several mechanisms:

- With increased anaerobic exercise, changes in the muscle-fiber population occur, resulting in more anaerobic fibers and fewer aerobic ones.

- With anaerobic exercise there is much more lactic acid produced compared to any other activity. This can inhibit the enzymes necessary for the aerobic fibers to function properly.

- Eating too much carbohydrate, especially refined sugar, increases sugar-burning and decreases fat-burning.

- Because of the influence on the sympathetic nervous system, too much anaerobic exercise results in increased adrenal-stress hormone. For many people, any amount of anaerobic exercise is too much. But you don't need anaerobic exercise to trigger stress. Work stress, for example, can produce the same anaerobic stress (albeit without muscle stimulation) and aerobic inhibition.

It's possible to improve both aerobic and anaerobic function, with the result of high levels of both. The first step is improving your aerobic system. Since the human body is made up of mostly aerobic muscle fibers, most of your activity should be aerobic. Some people overuse their anaerobic systems when they should be encouraging aerobic function to accomplish the same tasks. From the time they get up in the morning until they finally drop back into bed at night, too many people are rushing, hurrying and under stress. We need to learn to better pace our lives, just as if we had a 1,000-mile journey to complete. Aerobic exercise, along with good nutrition and dietary factors, can correct this imbalance, allowing you to build better health.

### Case History
*Gary, a high-level executive in a stressful job, started exercising at his company's gym. At first he felt great. He lifted weights three or four times a week, jogged on the treadmill and played squash. But after a few months his shoulder began hurting. Then his knee started to hurt and he felt tired much of the day. In my consultation and exam I found Gary to be in a state of anaerobic excess. He was placed on an easy aerobic walking program with some easy stationary cycling and swimming, and was asked to do no anaerobic exercise. Within three weeks, Gary was much*

*more energetic, and his shoulder and knee problems were gone. After*
*three months of building up his aerobic system, Gary was ready to add*
*weights to his routine.*

Gary had an aerobic deficiency and an anaerobic excess, which is common. He had to do two things to improve his fitness and health. First, he had to stop all anaerobic exercise. By doing this, the potential inhibiting stress was taken off the aerobic system. Second, he had to develop his aerobic system. In Gary's case, it took three months to build his aerobic system to a level that was balanced with his anaerobic system. Only then could he return to anaerobic work.

The time necessary to develop the aerobic system is sometimes referred to as building an aerobic base. To do this efficiently, it takes time, about three months minimally, or for many people, up to six months or more. It takes discipline to not go anaerobic when working out, and to pay attention to all lifestyle factors related to improving the aerobic system.

### Anaerobic Exercise and Wasting Disease

Some people obtain important benefits from lifting weights or performing other hard anaerobic exercise, when performed for short periods such as three to four weeks. However, for most people, ongoing anaerobic exercise creates a body chemistry similar to cancer, HIV or other wasting diseases.

One of the more frustrating issues I faced in practice was trying to convince many people that their exercise program was literally running them into the ground — that they were sacrificing health for fitness. Unfortunately, I found this difficult to discuss with most people, except for scientists (probably because so much of the information comes from published scientific studies).

Studies show that the biochemical patterns seen in certain disease states such as cancer and HIV infection are similar to patterns found in healthy people who performed anaerobic exercise three times a week for one hour over a four- to eight-week period. These similar unhealthy states include low amino acids (glutamine and cysteine), low T-cell counts (immune system function) and the loss of lean body tissue (muscle). Even in those who lost weight, it was found that most of what was lost was muscle, not fat. These same problems were not observed in aerobic exercisers.

Oxidative stress is also associated with anaerobic training and a variety of diseases. The significant production of oxygen free radicals can cause damage to virtually all bodily systems. This significantly increases the need for all types of antioxidants. Since the average person who performs anaerobic exercises may not get sufficient antioxidant nutrients from the diet, and most supplements are not complete in their antioxidant components, harmful free-radical damage is very common.

The real game with anaerobic exercise is to balance the workouts with the right nutritional components. The majority of a yearly program should be made up of aerobic exercise, with short periods (three to four weeks) of anaerobic training, if any. Most people — from casual exercisers to highly competitive athletes — can obtain tremendous benefits from aerobic activity with little or no need for anaerobic training. On the dietary and nutritional side, be sure to eat enough protein to meet the needs for glutamine, cysteine and other amino acids, with fresh vegetables and fruits for antioxidants, and take supplements if these nutrients are not obtained from the diet. For athletes, more details can be found in two of my books, *Eating for Endurance* and *Training for Endurance*.

### Lifting Weights? Do It Right

Weight-lifting can help you maintain strength and muscle mass, especially as you age. But incorporating this type of anaerobic training into an overall healthy conditioning program can be tricky. Lifting weights primarily stimulates anaerobic muscle fibers.

Recent studies have shown that too much ongoing anaerobic exercise, including weight-lifting, produces a body chemistry similar to that seen in cancer and AIDS patients. Anaerobic exercise is a tremendous stress on the body that can lead to many problems if overdone. Most injuries occur in overworked anaerobic muscle fibers or are due to weak aerobic muscle fibers, both often a direct result of too much anaerobic activity. In addition, anaerobic exercise such as weight-lifting increases inflammation and the production of oxygen free radicals, both of which are associated with illness and disease. If you currently lift weights and have recurring illness, injury or other problems, it's time to re-evaluate your workout.

Start your weight-training program by doing none at all. First build a strong aerobic base through walking, jogging, running, cycling or other aerobic activity before introducing anaerobic activity. Use the 180 Formula and MAF Test as described in the next chapter.

Once your aerobic system is ready to handle anaerobic exercise, you must determine how much it can handle. Everyone is different, and stress from other areas in life also stresses the anaerobic system. For some people one anaerobic workout per week is sufficient; others with low-stress lifestyles may be able to handle up to three weekly anaerobic workouts.

Regardless, the bulk of benefits will be gained in three to four weeks, at which point it's time to focus again on the aerobic system. In this way you will be able to reap the benefits of anaerobic training with less chance for illness, injury or compromised body chemistry.

# 24 Taking the Guesswork Out of Exercise: Heart-Rate Monitoring

As important as it is to keep most workouts aerobic, most people do just the opposite. Instead of programming their bodies to burn fat and spare sugar, they are developing their anaerobic systems to burn more sugar, and less fat. Performing aerobic exercise is a key to developing the aerobic system. You can walk, jog, run, bike, swim, dance or do almost anything aerobically. Unfortunately, you can also do these activities anaerobically.

How can you be sure your exercise is aerobic? In chapter 2 I talked about measuring oxygen and carbon dioxide during exercise to determine the respiratory quotient (RQ), which indicates how much fat and sugar a person is burning. As accurate as this may be, it is also very impractical for everyday use. The most useful and least expensive way to check your exercise level is with a heart-rate monitor.

Many people now use heart-rate monitors while running, walking, dancing or riding a bike. This takes the guesswork out of exercise — if you know what to look for. As you attain higher levels of exercise intensity, less fat and more sugar is burned for energy. Most importantly, the level of exercise intensity will dictate how your body reacts to that exercise session during the next 24 hours. Higher levels of intensity program your body to burn more sugar and less fat, and easier exercise does just the opposite. You can monitor the type of programming your body gets by checking your heart rate.

There are two ways to check your heart rate, by hand or using a monitor. Trying to monitor your heart rate by stopping to take your pulse is often not very accurate. If you are just one or two beats off in a six-second count, that's a difference of 10 to 20 beats per minute! When you stop to take a pulse, your heart rate decreases rapidly. In six seconds, the rate may drop by 10, 15 or 20 beats per minute. In addition, even the light pressure used to take your pulse from the carotid artery in the neck can trigger a more rapid slowing of the heart rate. Besides getting an inaccurate count, you run the risk of fainting. An accurate heart-monitoring device is the answer to these problems.

Basic heart-rate monitors employ a strap around the lower chest. They sense the heart rate by picking up vibrations of the heartbeat through the ribs. The heart rate is then transmitted to a watch worn on the wrist. Many monitors also have an alarm that sounds when you exercise above or below your individually set heart rate.

There are also devices that measure distal pulses. These include monitors with sensors that attach to your fingertip or earlobe to pick up pulses. They are less accurate and not as convenient to use for walking or jogging, but may be useful for working on a stationary apparatus, such as a bike.

According to *Dorland's Medical Dictionary*, biofeedback is visual or auditory evidence to a person of the status of body function so that one may exert control over that function. Heart-rate monitors are used just like any other biofeedback device. They tell you what is going on inside your body.

As a student involved in a biofeedback research project, I measured responses in human subjects to various physiological inputs: sounds, visual effects and various physical stimulations, including exercise. The observed reactions were evaluated by measuring temperature, sweating and heart rate. It became evident that using the heart rate to objectively measure body function was simple, accurate and useful. Its application in exercise was obvious.

Early in my practice, in the late 1970s, I began using heart monitors to evaluate the quality of workouts done by patients. In time, by correlating these observations with actual RQ measurements of patients, I developed a method for determining the best heart rate to use for building the aerobic system more efficiently, and a test to determine if a person is really getting benefits from exercise. Let's discuss these very important aspects of developing maximum aerobic function, beginning with a formula I developed in the early 1980s.

### The 180 Formula

The first step in the ideal exercise program is to find what level of effort is best for you. There is an ideal heart rate, which, when not exceeded, will give you optimal aerobic benefits. Traditionally, this level has been determined one of two ways: with the talk test, or with the 220 formula. The *180 Formula* replaces both.

You may be familiar with the talk test, which assumes you are exercising within your aerobic range if you can comfortably talk to an exercise partner during a workout. This test is unreliable and in fact often maintains someone in a mild anaerobic state.

The 220 formula, which unfortunately is still widely used, has you subtract your age from 220 and multiply the difference by a figure ranging from 65 to 85 percent. The resulting number supposedly provides you with the training heart rate.

This formula contains two serious errors. It assumes that 220 minus your age is your maximum heart rate. In reality, most people who obtain their maximum heart rate by pushing themselves to exhaustion (I don't recommend you do this) will find it's probably not 220 minus their age. About a third find their maximum is above, a third will be below and only a third may be close to 220 minus their age.

The second inaccuracy is the multiplier, which can range between 65 to 85 percent. This arbitrary figure doesn't consider a person's overall health or fitness. Do you use 65 or 75 percent? How about 80 or 70 percent? Without a more precise indicator, you are leaving your fitness to chance. Most people opt for the no-pain, no-gain approach and guess at a number that offers a higher heart rate.

Rather than guess, it's best to use a formula that is not only more sensible, but has a proven success record and is more scientific: the 180 Formula. This method also considers physiological rather than just chronological age. To find your maximum aerobic exercise heart rate, first subtract your age from 180. Next, find the best category for your present state, as follows.

**Calculating Your Maximum Aerobic Heart Rate**

1. **Subtract your age from 180** (180 – age)

2. **Modify this number** by selecting one of the following categories:

   a. If you have, or are recovering from, a major illness (heart disease, any surgery or hospital stay, etc.) or if you are on any regular medication, **subtract 10.**

   b. If you have been exercising but have been injured or are regressing in your efforts (not showing much improvement), or if you often get colds or flu, or have allergies, or if you have not exercised before, **subtract 5.**

   c. If you have been exercising for up to two years at least four times a week without any injury, and if you have not had colds or flu more than once or twice a year, **subtract 0.**

   d. If you have been exercising for more than two years without any injury, have been making progress, and are a competitive athlete, **add 5.**

**183**

For example, if you are 30 years old and fit into category "b":

**180 – 30 = 150, then 150 – 5 = 145 beats per minute**

The result of the equation is your maximum aerobic heart rate. In this example, exercising at a heart rate of 145 beats per minute will be highly aerobic, allowing you to develop maximum aerobic function. Exercising at heart rates above this level will add a significant anaerobic component to the workout, and start to develop your anaerobic system, exemplified by a shift to more sugar-burning and less fat-burning. If you prefer to exercise below your maximum aerobic heart rate, you will still derive good aerobic benefits, but progress at a slightly slower pace.

The only exceptions for this formula are for people over the age of 65, and those under the age of 16, as follows:

- For seniors in category "c" or "d," you may have to add up to 10 beats after obtaining your maximum aerobic heart rate. That doesn't mean you *must* add 10 beats. This is such an individualized category, getting assistance from a professional would be very helpful. Note: it always pays to be conservative, so if your resulting number is lower, it's also safer compared to guessing it may be a higher number.

- For kids under the age of 16, there's no need to use the 180 Formula. Instead, use 165 as the maximum aerobic heart rate. Ideally, kids may be very intuitive, and may not even need heart monitors. Unfortunately, most have already been influenced by the no-pain, no-gain work ethic in sports. If this is the case, a monitor will help them.

When you first exercise at your maximum aerobic heart rate, it may seem too easy. Many people have told me initially they can't imagine it's worth the time. I tell them to not only imagine it will help, but to understand how the body really works.

In a short time, exercise will become more enjoyable, and you'll find more work is needed to maintain your heart rate. In other words, as your aerobic system builds up, you'll need to walk, ride or dance faster to attain your maximum aerobic heart rate. If you're a runner, your minute-per-mile pace will get faster; bikers will ride at higher miles per hour at the same heart rate; and so on.

**Case History**

*Sally was very dedicated to her exercise routine. She went to aerobic dance class four mornings a week, and walked twice weekly with friends. But her time was not well spent, she thought, since her weight and body fat didn't change much in the two years she worked out. She also was very tired on the days she did aerobics. I asked Sally to wear a heart monitor during her aerobics class and when she walked. Not surprisingly, her heart rate exceeded 180 beats per minute during aerobics, and averaged 155 on her walks. But Sally's maximum aerobic heart rate was 140. Thus she had programmed her body to burn more sugar and less fat.*

*After seeing that she couldn't physically perform the aerobic routine during an advanced class without her heart rate going over 140, Sally went to an easier class where she was able to control her heart rate at 140. She also began walking on her own, at a much slower pace. Within a couple of months, Sally lost more weight than in the previous two years, and her workouts now gave her energy. In time she was able to go back to the advanced aerobics class and walk with her friends while maintaining a 140 heart rate.*

Once you find your maximum aerobic heart rate, you can conveniently make a range that starts 10 beats below that number. Most heart-rate monitors can be set for your range, providing you with an audible indication if your heart rate goes over or under your preset levels. Set yours at the maximum aerobic rate you determined. Most monitors also provide for a low setting, which could be 10 below the high. This gives you a comfortable range. For example, if your maximum aerobic heart rate is 145, then the low would be 135; set the monitor for a range between 135 and 145.

It's not absolutely necessary to work out in your range — you just don't want to exceed it. If you're more comfortable exercising under that range, you will still derive good aerobic benefits.

## Applying the 180 Formula

The 180 Formula applies to all activities. At the same heart rate, different types of exercise require about the same levels of metabolic activity. So whether you're swimming, biking or walking, many physiological parameters are the same.

One significant difference is the perceived exertion, a subjective feeling you have about how easy or hard the workout seems. Running at a heart rate of 140, for example, has a perceived exertion that's lower than swimming at that rate. That is, swimming at a 140 heart rate (given the same physical know-how) usually feels more difficult. This difference has to do with gravity stress. The gravity-stress difference between swimming and running is significant; there is very little gravity influence in the water, but gravity maximally affects your body during running. A lot of energy may not have to go into countering gravity stress in the pool but just the opposite is true during a run. Another way of looking at this phenomenon is that the heart rate during swimming is lower compared to running at the same effort, since the stress level is diminished in the water.

Riding a bike falls between the two extremes of swimming and running, along with cross-country skiing, skating and most other endurance activities. In these actions, there is some gravity stress along with mechanical stress.

Another factor that influences the heart rate is technique. For the beginning swimmer, the heart rate is usually much higher. As your technique improves, the stress level decreases and the same intensity results in lower heart rates. You need to swim faster to maintain your maximum aerobic heart rate.

The benefits of training with a heart monitor are many, and only with time and experience will you come to truly appreciate them. Specifically, a significant benefit of applying the 180 Formula to heart-rate exercise is the body's chemical response to exercise at a relatively lower level of intensity. Normally, the body produces oxygen free radicals in response to many stresses, including anaerobic exercise. Too many of these free radicals contribute to degenerative problems such as inflammatory conditions, heart disease and cancer. Increased free radicals also speed the aging process. Exercising above your maximum aerobic level causes the body to produce large amounts of free radicals, even if you're only a little above the level. Using the 180 Formula as your guide minimizes free-radical production. Studies show that training at this efficient intensity is ideal when free-radical stress is a concern.

**The MAF Test**
Another important benefit of using a heart-rate monitor is the ability to objectively measure your aerobic progress. This is accomplished using the Maximum Aerobic Function Test, or *MAF Test*.

The MAF Test objectively measures the improvements you make in the aerobic system. Without objective measurements, you can fool yourself into thinking all is well with your exercise. More importantly, the MAF Test tells you if you're headed in the wrong direction, either from too much anaerobic exercise, too little aerobic exercise or any imbalance that is having an adverse effect on the aerobic system.

The MAF Test can be performed using any exercise except weight-lifting. During the test use your maximum aerobic heart rate found with the 180 Formula. While working out at that heart rate, determine some parameter such as your walking, jogging or running pace (in minutes per mile), cycling speed (miles per hour) or repetitions (laps in a pool) over time. The test can also be done on stationary equipment such as a stair stepper or other apparatus that measures output.

If you want to test your maximum aerobic function during walking, for example, go to the high-school track and walk at your maximum aerobic heart rate. Determine how long it takes to walk one mile at this heart rate. Record your time in a diary or on your calendar. If you normally walk two or three miles, you can record each mile. It is normal for the times to get slower as the miles accumulate.

Below is an actual example of an MAF Test performed by walking on a track, at a heart rate of 145, calculating time in minutes per mile:

**Mile 1**  16:32 (16 minutes and 32 seconds)
**Mile 2**  16:46
**Mile 3**  17:09

During any one MAF Test, your times should always get slower with successive repetitions. In other words, the first mile should always be the fastest, and the last the slowest. If that's not the case, it usually means you haven't warmed up enough, as discussed in a following chapter.

The MAF Test should indicate faster times as the weeks pass. This means the aerobic system is improving and you're burning more fat, enabling you to do more work with the same effort. Even if you walk or run longer distances, your MAF Test should show the same progression of results, providing you heed your maximum aerobic heart rate. Below is an example showing the improvement of the same person from above:

|  | September | October | November | December |
|---|---|---|---|---|
| **Mile 1** | 16:32 | 15:49 | 15:35 | 15:10 |
| **Mile 2** | 16:46 | 16:06 | 15:43 | 15:22 |
| **Mile 3** | 17:09 | 16:14 | 15:57 | 15:31 |

Performing the MAF Test on a bike is similar. On your bike you have a couple of effective ways to record the test. When riding outside, the easiest method is to pick a bike course that initially takes about 30 minutes to complete. Following a warm-up, ride at your maximum aerobic heart rate, and record exactly how long it takes to ride the test course. As you progress, your times should get faster. Riding your course today, for example, may take 30 minutes and 50 seconds. In three weeks it may take you 29:23 and in another three weeks 27:35. After three months of base work, the same course may take you 26 minutes flat.

Another option is to ride on a flat course and see what pace you can maintain while holding your heart rate at your max aerobic level. This works best on a stationary apparatus. As you progress, your miles-per-hour should increase. If you start at 12 mph, for example, following a three-month aerobic base you might be riding 17 mph at the same heart rate.

Perform the MAF Test regularly, throughout the year, and chart your results. I recommend doing the test every three or four weeks. Testing yourself too often may result in obsession. Usually, you won't improve significantly within one week.

For those who walk, or do other activities that, over time, will not raise the heart rate to the maximum aerobic level, it's possible to do the MAF Test without using the maximum aerobic heart rate. Since it's usually too difficult to reach that heart rate, choose a lower rate for your MAF Test. For example, if you have difficulty reaching 150, your max aerobic rate, use 125 during your walk as the rate for your MAF Test.

Performing the test irregularly or not often enough defeats one of its purposes — knowing when your aerobic system is getting off course. One of the great benefits of the MAF Test is its ability to objectively inform you of an obstacle long before you feel bad or get injured. If something interferes with your progress, such as exercise itself, diet, or stress, you don't want to wait until you're feeling bad or gaining weight to find that out.

### Phases of Aerobic Function

An important element of the MAF Test is knowing what is normal and what isn't. During the course of your program, you could encounter three different phases: progression, plateau and regression.

When you successfully develop your aerobic system, you will have more energy and better aerobic function, as indicated by your MAF Test. This is the progressive phase, and it can and should continue for many years without regression. As you improve, further progression will happen more slowly. For example, the first year your walking may improve from 18 minutes to 13 minutes per mile. The second year, your improvement may only go from 13 minutes per mile, walking, to 10 minutes per mile, jogging.

There will be periods of plateaus. Actually, there are two different kinds of plateaus, one normal and the other unhealthy. With improvement, you will eventually arrive at a normal leveling off — almost as if your body needs a rest from the progress it's making. The metabolic, neurological and muscular aspects of the body require a period of adjustment, and the body may need some time for a recovery. These normal plateaus shouldn't last too long, perhaps a few weeks to a few months. Then, progress should resume, as measured by the MAF Test. If you stay in your plateau for longer periods, it may be abnormal.

An abnormal plateau is due to some obstacle that prevents progress. The MAF Test can help diagnose an abnormal plateau. Once your test has stayed the same for too long, the next step is to find out why. There could be many factors.

By far the most common reason for an abnormal plateau is stress. Remember, stress can be physical, chemical or mental. Typically, some lifestyle stress or stresses could cause your aerobic system to plateau. The weather may also be a stress that can halt progression.

If you think your plateau is abnormal, assess yourself carefully, or get help from a professional. Other common problems include too much exercise (especially the anaerobic type), dehydration, poor diet and nutritional problems. These factors are discussed in detail in this book.

Even worse than not making progress is regressing. Indeed, that's just what happens if your plateau is prolonged. An abnormal plateau will eventually cause your MAF Test to get worse each time you check it. If this happens, your body is in a "red alert" and you should be very cautious. This is when you become most vulnerable to injury and ill health. One recommended strategy is to cut your overall exercise time by 50 percent until you find the problem. This will at least ensure you get more rest and recovery. If you don't respect the advice of your body, you may ultimately need to seek first-aid advice from a professional. Exhaustion, injury, illness or some other major breakdown, possibly including mental breakdown, can occur.

## Be Consistent

There are a number of factors that may affect your MAF Test results. When walking, for example, the type of track surface may have a slight influence on your pace. The modern high-tech track surfaces result in a slightly faster pace, whereas the old cinder and dirt tracks will slow your pace at the same heart rate. Uneven tracks will give slower times compared to perfectly flat surfaces.

On your bike, the roughness of the road surface, varying grades and traffic can affect your test results. Hills usually result in a slowing of pace, unless there are significantly more downhills. A good option is to use a stationary apparatus on your test days.

To ensure the MAF Test is accurate, be consistent; use the same course or method each time you test yourself. If you change your test course, be sure to note it in your diary or chart.

Other factors that could affect your test include weather conditions such as wind, rain, snow, temperature and humidity; altitude; hydration; and your equipment. Most of these factors can work against you by increasing your physical effort, which raises the heart rate. Since you are working at a specific heart rate, the result is a slower pace.

One other factor worth mentioning is ill health. When you are sick, your body's immune system is working hard to recover, and it needs all the energy it can get. The last thing your body wants to do at this time is work out, especially when you have an elevated temperature. Don't exercise if you are ill. If you've ever attempted it and worn a heart monitor, you know what happens: your heart rate elevates, sometimes drastically. The same effect is observed if you are anemic: less oxygen can be delivered to the muscles, and your tests will worsen.

By using the 180 Formula and regularly performing the MAF Test you will be on the right road for improving health and fitness. But there's one thing missing — in order for you to gain fitness, you need to use these tools within the context of a regular exercise routine. The next chapters offer suggestions for how you can develop a lasting exercise program for a lifetime of health and fitness.

# 25 The Real Warm-Up and Cool-Down

Most people think that warming up means stretching. This isn't true. A real warm-up provides many important benefits, most of which stretching can't give. What's more, stretching can often do more harm than good.

Warming up is the first step of exercise; it's the slow shifting of blood into the working muscles. The key word is *slow*. Shifting the blood into the muscles too quickly can be a significant stress on the rest of the body. Specifically, the blood going into the muscles comes from other important areas of the body including the nervous system, adrenal glands and intestines. Diverting the blood out of these areas and circulating it into the muscles too quickly can be much like going into shock. When a warm-up is done slowly, the organs and glands can properly compensate for this normal activity. Warming up provides three important benefits:

- It increases the blood flow, bringing oxygen and nutrients into the muscles, and removing waste products.

- It increases the fats in the blood that are used for muscle energy.

- It increases flexibility in all the joints by gently lengthening the muscles.

The warm-up can be any easy, low-heart-rate activity. Begin your exercise by slowly raising your heart rate from its starting point of say, 75 bpm. Slowly elevate the heart rate, over a 12- to 15-minute period, arriving at your maximum aerobic level only after 15 minutes. At this point, you can maintain your maximum aerobic heart rate until nearing the end of your workout, when you begin to cool down.

## The Cool-Down

The final 12 to 15 minutes of your workout are also important; it's vital to slowly re-establish nearly normal circulation without "pooling" blood in the muscles. You want to re-establish the normal circulation in the organs and glands to begin the 24-hour process of recovery and obtaining the benefits from your exercise. This slow lowering of the heart rate from the maximum aerobic level back to near-resting level is called the cool-down.

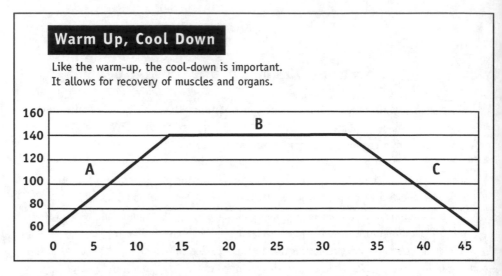

The graph above shows heart-rate changes in relation to time for
**A:** Warming up, **B:** Maintaining the maximum aerobic level, and **C:** Cooling down.

### Stretching and Flexibility

From your earliest years in school you were probably taught to stretch before exercising. Even people who don't work out sometimes think stretching is a good way to get rid of body aches and pains and so-called tight muscles. Go to any fitness center and you'll see that many people do it. Many think if they can touch their toes, they're fit.

There's very little, if any, scientific information demonstrating that static stretching is beneficial, especially the way most people do it. As a matter of fact, there's quite a bit of evidence showing it's harmful.

One of the most common reasons people give for stretching is injury prevention. But studies show static stretching can actually increase the risk of injury! One of many examples given is the hamstring muscles. It is both the most frequently injured muscle group and the most stretched.

Many people need flexibility, and I often recommend that increases in flexibility be made to prevent injury and create a more stable physical body. This increased flexibility can be accomplished with a proper warm-up, rather than with stretching. Even patients with arthritis can improve flexibility with an easy aerobic warm-up of 15 minutes, and be as flexible as if they had stretched, without the risk. Before addressing the potential dangers, I'd like to talk about the two different kinds of stretching, referred to as static and ballistic.

### Static Stretching

Static stretching is a very slow, deliberate movement, lightly stretching a muscle and holding it unchanged for up to 30 seconds. When properly done, this activity promotes relaxation of the muscle fibers being stretched. Optimal static stretching requires that each muscle group throughout the body be sequentially repeated three to four times. It also demands that the activity be done slowly. Note some of the key words: slow, deliberate, lightly stretch. And also note the need to stretch each muscle group three to four times. All this takes time, which most people just don't think they have or don't make time for.

There are two different types of static stretching: active and passive. Active stretching is safer than passive. Active stretching is accomplished by contracting the antagonist muscle (the one opposite the muscle you're stretching). For example, to actively stretch the hamstring muscles, the quadriceps are contracted.

Passive stretching uses either gravity or force by another body part or person to move a body segment to the end of its range of motion or beyond — the reason this form of stretching can so easily cause injury. We sometimes see football players stretching one leg by having another player lean on it.

### Ballistic Stretching

The second basic type of stretching is called ballistic. This is a "bouncing" method and is the most common type done by both beginners and seasoned exercisers. It makes use of the body's momentum to repeatedly stretch a joint position to or beyond the extreme ranges of motion. Because this method is more rapid than static stretching, it activates the stretch reflex, which increases tension in the muscle, rather than relaxation. This can result in micro-tearing of muscle fibers with resultant injury. Ballistic stretching is the type most people say they don't do, but really are doing. That's because most people are in a hurry when stretching.

Flexibility refers to the relative range of motion allowed at a joint. This is related to the tension in the muscles around the joint, those that move or restrict the joint. The risk of injury is increased when:

• Joint flexibility is increased too much.

• Joint flexibility is greatly diminished.

• An imbalance in joint flexibility exists between left and right (or front and back) sides of the body.

When it comes to flexibility, don't assume more is better. A study of U.S. Army recruits found the least flexible and the most flexible were more than twice as likely to get injured compared to those whose joints had moderate flexibility.

People who stretch generally are injured more often than those who don't stretch. That's been my observation during more than 20 years of treating patients, and the opinion and observation of many other professionals in all fields. In addition, scientific studies support our observations.

J.P. Halbertsma and L.N. Goeken, in a study of men and women 20 to 38 years of age with tight and stiff hamstrings, state that "stretching exercises do not make short hamstrings any longer or less stiff."

Richard Dominguez, an orthopedic surgeon at Loyola University Medical Center and author, also disapproves of stretching. "Flexibility should not be a goal in itself, but the result of . . . training. Strengthening the muscles around a joint naturally increases flexibility. If you can bend a joint beyond your ability to control it with muscle strength, you risk either tearing the muscles, tendons or ligaments that support the joint, or damaging the joint through abnormal pressure on it." Among the specific stretches Dominguez says are most damaging are the yoga plow, hurdler's stretch, toe touching and the stiff-leg raise. The types of injury created by stretching aren't associated with just the muscle being stretched. The tendons and ligaments associated with that muscle, and even the joint controlled by that muscle, are at risk.

There's also a chemical factor to consider. Repetitive exercise, such as walking, swimming, biking and other activities, results in the production of chemicals that increase inflammation. Adding stretching increases the potential for even more inflammation.

Many athletes stretch to help performance. But studies show static stretching doesn't improve athletic performance and may actually hinder it. For those who require a wider range of motion, stretching may be necessary. These include dancers, sprinters and gymnasts, but usually not most people doing aerobic exercise.

### Case History

*Randy began his morning with 10 minutes of stretching. The first 15 minutes of his bike workout was spent riding up hills from his house out of the valley. When he first used a heart monitor, his rate surged to 180 within five minutes. Randy couldn't imagine how any of that was related to his low-back pain. But by performing manual muscle testing, we discovered that Randy's hamstring muscles were overstretched, and therefore were not helping to support his low back. The first recommendation was to stop stretching his already overstretched hamstrings. Within a couple of weeks Randy's low-back pain improved. This was followed by the difficult task of adjusting his morning ride to include a warm-up, and to avoid going directly to the hills, with the resultant high heart rate. The solution was for Randy to ride indoors on a stationary apparatus for about 15 minutes before going outside, then riding very slowly until getting past the hills. When he was able to accomplish this, both his back pain and his chronic asthma disappeared.*

## Whole-Body Flexibility

Yoga and other "whole-body" flexibility activities are very different from stretching as I've described it above. When properly done, in a very slow, deliberate and easy motion, whole-body flexibility activities are healthy, safe and very effective. They're also recommended as a source of relaxation and meditation. If you wish to learn yoga or other flexibility activities find a course or an instructor who won't rush the sessions or push you beyond your limits. Don't attend if you can't put in the appropriate amount of time, and never go beyond your needs. Too many people try to rush into yoga positions that normally take a long time to establish.

While many people think they are doing the right thing by stretching, they would be better served by properly warming up and cooling down before exercising. For those who still wish to improve flexibility and who have the time to do it right, yoga is the best choice.

# 26 Your Exercise Program

It's clear that regular aerobic exercise is essential for you to attain the full bene-fits of better human performance. But I want to re-emphasize that I'm not talk-ing about a no-pain, no-gain exercise program that will fall by the wayside as quickly as you start it. Instead I am talking about incorporating into your lifestyle an ongoing, long-term natural aerobic exercise program that will greatly improve your energy levels, stamina and endurance, while helping you tone the aerobic muscles and train your body to burn more fat for energy. Your exercise routine should be something that you look forward to continuing for a lifetime.

As discussed, aerobic exercise differs greatly from anaerobic exercise such as fast running, weight-lifting and most "aerobics" classes. In fact, aerobics classes are often anaerobic exercise due to the intensity at which they are con-ducted. You now know the main difference between aerobic and anaerobic exer-cise is that aerobic exercise uses more fat as a fuel while anaerobic exercise uses more sugar. Moreover, when you perform aerobic exercise, you program your body to burn more fat as a fuel for all your activities, from working to sleeping. Anaer-obic exercise programs, on the other hand, train your body to burn more sugar and less fat throughout your day.

It's up to you to decide what type of aerobic activity and how much of it you want to do. For most people, a variety of activities works best. Exercise programs are quite individual. Some people just want to stay fit and healthy, and keep their weight in check. Others have goals like winning the Ironman Triathlon. For either of these types, and for everyone in between, many basic principles are the same. All people who exercise want to gradually build up to a specific level, using the 180 Formula as discussed in chapter 24, to improve aerobic fitness. Additionally, anyone on an exercise plan needs to balance this program with everything else in his or her life, including proper rest and recovery. Finally, it's important that you properly warm up and cool down before exercising as dis-cussed in the last chapter.

### Walking Your Way to Fitness and Health

Of all the types of exercise, walking is the one I recommend the most, and not just for beginners, but for regular exercisers and even professional athletes. It's the most fail-safe exercise. Scientific studies show that walking burns a higher percentage of fat than any other activity because of its low intensity. Walking activates the small aerobic muscle fibers, which often are not stimulated by high-er-intensity aerobic workouts. Walking also helps circulate blood, process lactic acid and improve lymph drainage (important to the body's waste-removal system).

Walking is one of the best ways to get started on an exercise program since it's a simple, low-stress workout that is not easily overdone. Walkers gener-ally have little difficulty keeping their heart rates from getting too high, though there are exceptions. If there's a problem with walking, it's that the heart rate won't go high enough into the maximum aerobic range (which isn't absolutely necessary). The mechanics of walking result in less gravity stress than you experi-ence jogging or running, but still enough to give you the important bone-strengthening effects.

We've all heard and read about the many wonderful benefits of exercise. But did you know most studies that demonstrate these great benefits were done using walking? You don't need to make exercise complicated, expensive or intense. And I'm talking about just an easy walk — not power walking, race walking or carrying weights. Here are some of the facts about the benefits of easy walking:

- Regular, easy walking increases life expectancy. It also helps older adults maintain their functional independence, an important concern for society. Currently, the average number of non-func-tional years in our elderly population is about 12. That's a dozen years at the end of a lifespan of doing nothing: unable to care for yourself, walk, be productive or just enjoy life.

- Regular, easy physical exercise can help prevent and manage coronary heart disease, the leading cause of death in the United States, as well as hypertension, diabetes, osteoporosis and depression. This occurs through improved balance of blood fats, better clotting factors, improved circulation and the ability to more efficiently regulate blood sugar.

- Regular exercise decreases your risk of developing degenerative disease. The lack of exercise places more people at risk for coro-nary heart disease than all other risk factors. Aerobic deficiency is an independent risk factor for coronary heart disease, doubling the risk. Inactivity is almost as great a risk for coronary heart dis-ease as cigarette smoking and hypertension.

- Walking is associated with a lower rate of colon cancer, stroke and low-back injury.

All this can be accomplished with easy aerobic exercise. How easy? The equivalent of a sustained 30-minute walk, four or five times a week. Less than 30 percent of Americans are this active, including children who spend most of their spare time watching TV.

For some people, especially those who have been very inactive, even walking may pose overexercise problems. Whether 18 or 80, if you're beginning an exercise program, or have been inactive for a period of time and now want to start walking, consider using a heart monitor to take the guesswork out of your walk. I've seen too many beginners walking with too high a heart rate. It's often because they're with other people and the instinct to be competitive comes into play. Talking while walking also increases the heart rate, and so does walking up a hill too fast before some level of fitness has been achieved. Formerly athletically fit individuals seeking to restore their fitness can benefit from walking; it keeps them from being too aggressive early in their programs. The most important thing for a walker to realize is that it's a fat-burning and endurance routine. Don't worry about speed; instead, concern yourself with endurance. Base your walking on time rather than miles.

### Case History

*Dave, a former college All-American, was in his middle-40s, overweight and feeling the effects of work stress. Since he was in the athletic-apparel business, he wanted to appear more fit. He began walking on the high-school track almost every evening. He got out of breath and tired easily, so he kept his pace relatively slow. After a couple of months with virtually no results, Dave asked for help. I told him to perform his walk as he usually does, but with a heart monitor. To our surprise, his heart rate exceeded 170 and stayed there for nearly the entire workout. Once Dave began using a heart monitor regularly and kept his rate at the prescribed level of 130, it was only a couple of weeks before he felt some positive results. And within a couple of months, Dave was thinner, had more energy and was walking faster.*

### Walking for the Non-Walking Competitor

Walking is also valuable to the competitive athlete whose sport may be cycling, running or any other more intense aerobic or anaerobic activity.

Walking can be used as part of a warm-up and cool-down. Competitive athletes, when they're in a rush or working out with others, often don't warm up and cool down enough or properly. One way to ensure this is done is to walk for 5 or 10 minutes before each workout. Even if you bike or swim, a walk is a good way to warm up. The same is true for cooling down. When you get off your bike or get out of the pool, go for an easy walk to cool down. If you make it a habit, you won't feel right missing it.

Besides the cross-training effect on your muscles and nervous system, walking helps train muscle fibers you might not normally use in your workout. These are the very small aerobic fibers used during low-intensity activity. Many trained athletes say their weekly walk initially made them sore. That's due to the lack of use of these small muscle fibers, which also help break down lactic acid and bring more blood to the anaerobic fibers.

**Walking as a Therapy**

Walking is useful as therapy following an injury or a period in which you have decreased your workouts for any reason. If you're injured, you may be unable to run or ride but have no trouble walking. Doing an easy aerobic workout is much better than doing nothing. And walking is a good way to come back from a period of time off without throwing your body back into high-level workouts.

Sometimes, even walking is difficult due to an injury or some other problem. Try walking in a pool in waist- or chest-high water. Gradually walk in shallower water before trying it on dry land.

As great as walking can be, many people feel uncomfortable about doing it. They somehow feel it's not enough of a workout, or it's too easy. It's that no-pain, no-gain feeling your nervous system has recorded in its memory. It's time to add some new memory.

**Balanced Health and Fitness**

Working out adds many new dimensions to your life. The most positive are increased health and fitness. On the other end of the continuum is the stress of maintaining a regimen, and worse yet, the stress of overdoing it. Much like diet and nutrition, each person must find an individualized program to meet his or her particular needs. So start out as simply as possible. Then consider joining a group to get some psychological encouragement, as long as you can exercise within your own limits. Through this habit change, the exercise program becomes a positive addiction. Your routine will ultimately become a part of your day, like brushing your teeth.

There are a number of important factors to consider when starting or modifying your exercise routine:

- **Scheduling.** Create a realistic schedule of exercise that fits in with family, work and your other commitments. This will allow you to be more consistent, and help make it part of a new lifestyle.

- **Physical factors.** Be sure you can withstand the minor stress of exercise. Do you have some physical imbalances that may be aggravated by exercise? Take into consideration a history of prior injuries or conditions. Consider your workout surface — blacktop, wood and carpet are preferable to concrete, marble and steel. Grass and dirt surfaces may be safe, but they also can be stressful if they are uneven or too soft.

- **Chemical factors.** The proper nutrients, especially fats, are necessary for aerobic efficiency. High-sugar foods and drinks can be detrimental when consumed before workouts. Proper hydration is a must; drink water all day, not just after working out.

- **Psychological factors.** Studies have shown that people who exercise in the morning find it easier to maintain a regular program. But whether you exercise in the morning, midday or evening, be consistent. Write out a simple exercise program, if necessary. You are more apt to follow something you can see. Keep a log on a calendar or in a diary to see your success as the days, weeks and months go by.

- **Goals.** Set realistic goals. Some people merely want to progress to exercising 30 minutes a day. Be conservative, but don't hesitate to dream. Running a marathon after six months of training may be realistic only for very disciplined people who can control their stress. You won't break any records, and completing the marathon should be your only goal. I've worked with many patients who successfully, and in a healthy way, met that goal.

- **Habit change.** Starting an exercise program is, first of all, a change of habit. And as we all know, a habit change can be the most difficult change to make — even more difficult than the exercise itself. Generally, there are two barriers. One is just getting started and the other shows up two to four weeks later, when your enthusiasm wears off a bit. (Although being aware of this is usually incentive enough to keep you going.)

• **Time.** Most exercise should be measured in time, and not miles, laps or repetitions. At the onset, a minimal time is best, since the purpose initially is to develop an exercise habit. The only exception may be if you progress to anaerobic workouts, such as weight-lifting, where a range of measurements should always be used. This gives you more choice, allowing for daily fluctuations in energy level and time restraints. For example, when using weights, the number of repetitions may be 10 to 15, rather than "you must do 15 reps."

• **Intensity.** The intensity of your workout is an important consideration, as measured by the heart rate. Make sure you understand how to find your maximum aerobic heart rate using the 180 Formula, described in chapter 24. Base your exercise program on time and intensity (as per heart rate); e.g., 30 minutes of walking at a heart rate not to exceed 140 bpm, five times per week.

### A Word for Beginners

Even if you've never been active, aerobic exercise is easy and simple. If you are in reasonably good health and have no serious problems or injuries, it can be done with a simple 30-minute walk a minimum of four to five times per week. You can do this on your way to work, or on your way home, as part of your lunch break or anytime. It can be performed walking indoors or outdoors. Or you can use a treadmill or stationary bike, either in your home or at the gym. A simple aerobic workout will easily fit into your current work schedule and requires no special equipment, clothing or gear. Here is a typical starting program for a beginner:

• Thirty minutes easy walking.

• 12-minute warm-up period, 12-minute cool-down period.

• Heart rate not to exceed the maximum aerobic level.

• Monday through Friday schedule.

• Saturday and Sunday off.

Lack of time is no excuse for not exercising. You can always fit in a 30-minute workout at some point during the day. If you want, you can spend more than 30 minutes. Within that time, include a 12-minute warm-up period, where your activity level is very easy. For the next 6 minutes move at a faster pace, but not so fast that it becomes uncomfortable — there's no need to break a sweat and you should be able to carry on a conversation. The remaining 12 minutes is your cool-down, another period of very easy activity. This is an optimal aerobic workout — one you can do in your work clothes during the course of the day.

Remember, your basic beginning program should be tailored to your specific needs. While most people are capable of at least 30 minutes of walking, perhaps 45 minutes is a good starting point. The maximum starting point for any beginner is an hour. Still others may benefit starting with 20 minutes per session. If you are recovering from a chronic illness, or have been very inactive all your life, you should consider only 15 minutes of exercise, or even 10 minutes, as a start, and also consult your doctor.

### Case History

*Alice was about to celebrate her 50th birthday, and thought it was time to get into shape. She was never physically active in sports, although she raised four children. She began a simple program of walking for 20 minutes, Monday through Friday, taking Saturday and Sunday off. After two months, Alice was ready to increase to 30 minutes each day, and after another two months progressed to 45 minutes. After a couple of years, Alice had the desire to take a couple of long walks a week, gradually working up to about 90 minutes each time.*

How rapidly you increase the time period depends on your response. Whatever the starting point, assuming the proper time is chosen, maintain that time for at least three weeks. Listen to your body; it will tell you if and when you can increase. This is also true for any change: Maintain the new time for at least three weeks before increasing it if that's desired and there's no difficulty.

Don't increase more than 50 percent at any one time in a program of up to 45 minutes, and not more than 15 minutes when the program is 45 minutes or more. Some people are quite content remaining at 45 minutes. This is fine, since you can obtain many benefits when exercising at this level five times per week.

Perform the MAF Test every three to four weeks. If any problems develop, stop. A professional may be helpful in determining what's wrong.

What type of exercise should you do? When starting out, do almost anything, as long as it's aerobic. This may include, besides walking, riding a stationary bike, dancing, rebounding (trampoline), outdoor biking, swimming, hiking, cross-country skiing, and using various exercise machines, such as rowing and skiing. Jogging, or running, when done aerobically, is a healthy exercise. There is no universally accepted scientific distinction between running and jogging. For the purposes of this book, I refer to jogging when I mean a slower pace. Running occurs with progression and more speed, and involves a slightly different gait. Any combination of these activities is also acceptable, as long as your heart rate doesn't exceed your maximum aerobic level. If you wish, do two or three types of exercise throughout the week, or even in one workout. For example, you can walk for 15 minutes, ride a stationary bike for 20 minutes and dance for 15 minutes. This "cross-training" routine is actually healthier than doing just one exercise each session.

Anaerobic activities, including any type of weight-lifting, sit-ups, pushups or activities that raise the heart rate above your maximum aerobic heart rate are not acceptable substitutes for aerobic exercise. They shouldn't be started until after you have developed your aerobic system. For the beginner, my recommendation is to wait at least six months, and for those modifying their program, wait at least three to four months before performing any anaerobic work.

Tennis, racquetball and similar sports often end up being anaerobic for the beginner, because of the type of muscle fibers used and the high heart rates produced. They're fun to do, but should be considered "games" and not exercise unless they're performed regularly; e.g., if you walk four times per week, play tennis once a week, or 18 holes of golf once a week. In that case, a proper warm-up and cool-down is important, as well as regulating aerobic and anaerobic levels.

Once you have progressed through a certain number of weeks without any problems, you may want to further develop your health and fitness. The following section is for people who wish to take their fitness to another level.

**Progressive Fitness Programs**
To further increase your level of aerobic fitness, you may wish to spend more time at or just below your maximum aerobic heart rate. Be sure to pay close attention to your heart-rate monitor to make sure you are not going over the maximum. If you can't reach your maximum aerobic heart rate by walking, you can jog or run, or perform other activities. Other types of aerobic activity, such as biking, swimming or dancing, can also be used to improve your aerobic fitness. Be conservative, and begin this phase slowly.

### Case History

*Kelly didn't like jogging, but wanted to do a variety of exercises. After walking regularly for more than a year, she joined an aerobics class. She continued to wear her heart monitor, walking three days a week and going to aerobics three days. After a few months, when the weather turned cold, she bought a stationary bike and rode it instead of walking, only venturing outdoors to walk if the temperature was tolerable. In time, Kelly had no need for her heart monitor; she only was able to get her heart rate to about 130 despite her maximum aerobic level being 145 beats per minute. She still performed her MAF Test, but at a lower heart rate.*

Kelly was very happy maintaining her activity at this level. Some people may choose to go on and enjoy more serious workouts as follows.

### Basic Training

For many people, just exercising to be fit and healthy isn't enough. At some point in time this type of casual exercise program crosses over to a training program. Some people train to reach a certain goal, such as walking or running a certain distance or climbing a mountain. Others want to be competitive. If you wish to push your exercise program to this level, I recommend that you read *Training for Endurance*, which I wrote as a guide for those who are serious about improving their endurance. Here are some basic training guidelines for those who wish to go beyond casual exercise.

- Take at least one or two days off per week for rest and recovery.
- Once per week, if time allows, do two workouts in one day, preferably one in the morning and one in the evening. Both should be relatively easy, below the maximum aerobic level.
- Once per week, do one longer-than-normal workout.

If after several weeks of building aerobic base your MAF Tests are continuing to show improvement, you may wish to add some anaerobic activity. Many people benefit by performing some anaerobic activity, as long as the aerobic system is well developed first, though for some with a high stress level, maintaining an aerobic schedule throughout the year works well. Anaerobic exercise may include lifting light weights, faster running, jogging, dancing, biking, or anything that raises the heart rate higher than the aerobic maximum. The following factors should be considered when scheduling an anaerobic workout:

- For most, one or two anaerobic workouts per week is sufficient.

- Anaerobic workouts should never be on consecutive days.

- Anaerobic workouts should be preceded by a day off, or a short, easy aerobic day.

- Anaerobic workouts should be followed by a short, easy aerobic day.

- A warm-up and cool-down should surround anaerobic workouts.

- This anaerobic period should last no more than three to five weeks.

**Caution!**

Anaerobic exercise is a very common cause of injury, ill health and overtraining. It is also the most common reason so many who exercise have poorly functioning aerobic systems (and adrenal glands); they are anaerobic during many, if not most, of their exercise sessions. Be cautious when performing anaerobic workouts. Do your MAF Test during anaerobic periods. If you perform too much anaerobic work, you will know it by the results of your MAF Test.

Most people don't really need to do anaerobic workouts. Their lives have enough stresses that stimulate the neurological, metabolic and muscular systems to satisfy the minimal anaerobic requirements of the body. So don't be pressured into anaerobic workouts if you're not absolutely sure you want to.

An important rule is worth mentioning here again: Have fun in your workouts. If your exercise routine has become a stress, then something is wrong. Maybe it's time to change what you're doing. Maybe you shouldn't exercise with the people you're with. Whatever the case, if exercise isn't fun, find out why and correct it.

# 27 Work-Out Shoes: The Danger Underfoot

Just like finding the proper formula for nutrition and exercise, it's up to you to find the right shoes for your feet. That may sound simple, but the truth is most shoes — even the ones in the impressive television ads — can be hazardous to your health. Most modern exercise shoes offer too much support, are too heavy, and have too-thick soles. What's more, most people choose the wrong size. The result is a formula for injury.

Biomechanically incorrect shoes can cause physical stress throughout your body, and contribute to injury. Scientific studies show that the so-called protective features found in many shoes, including shock absorption and motion control, actually increase the likelihood of injury. For instance, some support systems can weaken your ankles, and soft, cushioned shoes can potentially lead to other injury. Furthermore, the thicker the sole, the more unstable your foot and ankle become.

Many of these oversupported shoes are also overweight. The seemingly insignificant weight added to your feet, in the course of the day or workout, produces large negative effects in the economy of locomotion. For example, for every 3 ounces of shoe weight, a 1 percent increase in oxygen uptake is required for the same performance.

The soles of your feet have millions of nerve endings that sense the pounding and stress of each step you take. This information is sent to the brain, which works together with your body to adapt to this stress by constantly adjusting your body during movement. This normal protective mechanism keeps you from accumulating excess wear and tear, and from being injured. When you cover the foot with a shoe, you risk interfering with this adaptive mechanism by preventing the nerve endings on the bottom of your feet from sensing and sending vital information to the brain. The result is a diminished ability by the foot and the rest of the body to adapt to normal activity, with potential damage to the ligaments, fascia, cartilage or bones in the foot. Because your feet are your foundation, any instability there could have dire consequences in the legs, knees, pelvis, low back or other areas. The impact that results from walking or training occurs whether a shoe is worn or not. Without a shoe, the body can adapt naturally. With a shoe, there may be interference in that adaptation process.

Barefoot is best because there is no interference with the nerves that sense contact with the ground. Overall, athletes who run barefoot are injured much less often than those who wear shoes. Unfortunately, this is not practical for most people, though you can still be barefoot whenever possible, such as in your home, or in your backyard. And if you live near a clean beach or a grassy area you can also do some barefoot walking or running on these surfaces.

### What to Wear?

The reality is that most people will have to wear shoes when going outside. When buying shoes, there are some things to consider. Look for shoes that are relatively flat and natural, ones that don't oversupport your foot or raise it off the ground too much. I often recommend the Wal-Mart Silver Series running shoe; some bigger shoe companies also are beginning to market shoes that are lower to the ground. In addition, some (not all) shoes called "racing flats" are built with less sole to come between your foot and the ground. Above all, forget the hype you hear about shoes. Consider the fact that one study of 5,000 runners showed that those using more-expensive running shoes with more shock-absorbing materials had a higher incidence of injury. It seems there is less chance of getting a running injury in less-expensive shoes. The main reason for wearing them is not support, but rather to protect your feet. This is another area of health in which getting assistance from a professional can help address your individual needs, especially if you have any problems with your feet, ankles or other areas affected by them.

In general, shoes with more cushioning are also likely to produce excessive pronation, an inward rotation of the foot. This is especially true of shoes with added soft midsole material. Excess heel height can also increase pronation, especially in shoes with heels that are thicker than about 1 inch. Too much heel height also causes the entire body to move abnormally.

Many shoe-support systems, including orthotics, can interfere with the normal functioning of the medial arch, the most important of three arches in the foot. I have only on rare occasions recommended orthotics, and only for a short time while the cause of the problem was being corrected.

Sorbothane and similar materials commonly used in exercise shoes and after-market insoles can also be counter-productive. While tests on machines demonstrate Sorbothane's great energy-absorbing abilities, a study on humans shows that insoles made of this material actually increase leg stress by 26 percent, enough to cause stress fractures.

Beware: The muscles of your foot and leg, especially the calf muscles, have adapted to the thickness of your shoe. If you suddenly change your shoe style by wearing flatter shoes, your muscles may have to re-adjust their length. This may take a couple of weeks, during which you may experience some calf discomfort.

### Case History

*Some time ago, after seeing running shoes get thicker, oversupported and softer, I thought about the times in college when I ran barefoot. From a practical standpoint, I wasn't willing to go that far, so I looked for the closest thing: a shoe that didn't restrict my natural foot and ankle mechanics but offered some protection from stones, and wear and tear. I started by looking at the newest exercise shoes but was immediately horrified at the prices. So I tried Keds. Yes, those cheap, no-attempt-at-support sneakers. For under $10, I was on my way. But my first day running left my calves quite sore. I realized it was just the difference in heel height, coming down to the ground from what seemed like stilts. The second day out, my legs wouldn't let me run. Even walking was uncomfortable. But I found walking on the treadmill acceptable to my body. After a week of that, and feeling better, I began running on the treadmill. And after another week, I ventured outside again. My calves adapted to the change in shoes and felt like those of a 20-year-old elite athlete once again. Unfortunately, Keds are no longer available in most men's sizes, but most women can find them.*

## Sizing Up Your Shoes

A significant number of people are wearing everyday, dress or exercise shoes that are too small. In addition to foot problems, this can cause pain or dysfunction in the ankle, leg, knee, hip, low back, and at times as high up as the neck or temporal mandibular (jaw) joint. And most often, the feet don't even hurt.

A study done in my clinic over an 18-month period found 52 percent of all new athletic patients were training in shoes that were too small. Once the problem was diagnosed, these patients usually required a change from one-half to one-and-one-half sizes larger. Another study by orthopedic surgeons showed that 88 percent of women wore everyday shoes that were too small.

### Case History

*Jim had seen eight different professionals for his problems. Because his symptoms were in both knees, most of their therapeutic attention was directed there. But it was Jim's shoes that told the real story. His right shoe had an area where the large toenail had worn through. Upon measuring his foot, it was found that his shoes were one entire size too small. "I thought they should be snug," he said. After wearing the correct-size shoes for a week, Jim was able to exercise painlessly for the first time in two-and-a-half years.*

You might think that the size of your feet is set by age 20, but that's not true. Normal size changes, as a result of changes in weight, muscular imbalance or pregnancy, occur regardless of age. Just being on your feet a lot can increase the size of your feet. This is due to the stretching or elongation of the ligaments and tendons, followed by a spreading of the bones in the foot. If you don't keep up with these changes by wearing larger-size shoes, you can create a major physical stress.

Wearing a shoe that's too small can cause a slow inward jamming of the toes, characteristically causing a backward subluxation of the first metatarsal joint, though any toe can be involved. This creates a mechanical instability in the foot which, if left uncorrected, can lead to other foot and ankle problems such as hammertoes and bunions. In time, the toes become spring-like; when a small shoe is slipped on, the toes spring in, and the tightness of the shoe is not obvious. The first metatarsal joint, however, is not as flexible as the joints of other toes, and therefore takes most of the abuse.

Due to the slow onset of this common problem, the first metatarsal jam is often asymptomatic; if you have it you usually don't complain of pain in that first toe joint. But visual examination of your feet will often reveal trauma, or micro-trauma (long-lasting mild stress) to the front of the toes. This often includes discoloration of the nail bed (a darkened toenail), blistering or callousing of the toes, or swelling of the first metatarsal joint (the "ball" of the foot). In more extreme cases, inspection of your shoe will reveal wear and tear, inside and out, as a result of the nail or front of the toe trying to push out of the shoe, sometimes causing a hole in the shoe.

Looking inside the shoe helps diagnose the problem. If you have a removable insole, take it out and study it. Look at the wear pattern (especially the indentation made from the toes), and see if the areas compressed by the toes are not completely on the insert, as they should be. Toes that overlap the top of the insert obviously indicate a too-small shoe.

The importance of proper-fitting shoes can't be overemphasized. Below are tips on finding an ideal-fitting shoe:

• Always measure your foot when buying shoes. After a certain age, many people don't have their feet measured when buying new shoes, since they don't realize their size could have changed. As a result, the same shoe size is worn for years, or even decades.

- Have both feet measured by a competent shoe-store salesperson, in a standing position on a hard floor. Do this at the end of the day, since most people's feet are slightly larger then, compared to the morning. (Of course, any meaningful daily size fluctuations must be differentiated from serious health problems, such as edema and certain pathological changes.) Use these sizes only as a gauge — the devices used for this measurement are consistent, but the sizes marked in the shoes aren't. A size 9 from one company may be more like an 8 from another. Don't buy shoes by their size but how they fit each foot. Even the same company may be very inconsistent when it comes to its own size standard.

- Spend adequate time trying on shoes in the store. Find a hard surface rather than the thick soft carpet in shoe stores, where almost any shoe will feel good. If there's no sturdy floor to walk on, ask if you can walk outside. If this is not allowed, shop elsewhere. Try on the size you think you normally wear. Even if that feels fine, try on a half-size larger. If that one feels the same, or even better, try on another half-size larger. Continue trying on larger half-sizes until you find the shoes that are obviously too large. Then go back to the previous half-size; usually that's the one that fits best. You may need to try different widths to get a perfect fit. Don't let anyone say you have to break them in before they feel good — the best shoes for you are the ones that feel good right away. Even though you may develop the reputation of being a nuisance at your shoe store, your body will benefit. While many salespeople are aware of how to find the right shoe size, many are not. Don't hesitate to educate them.

- For those who have a significant difference of more than a half-size between their two feet, fit the larger foot.

- Many women fit and function better in men's sports shoes than in women's. The first rule, though, is that the shoe must fit properly. Some women don't fit into men's shoes, and some stores don't carry men's shoes in sizes that are small enough.

- You may not find the right shoe in the first store you visit. Most outlets carry only a few of the many shoes in the marketplace. Often, shoes from mail-order outlets cost less. But be prepared to ship them back if they don't fit just right.

• Remember, manufacturers design new shoes based on trends of style, color and fancy gimmicks to market the shoe. That's why shoe styles come and go. If you find the shoe that fits perfectly, buy several pairs. Just be sure to try them all on, since the same shoe style may vary in size.

Some patients I worked with bought larger shoes after their initial problem was diagnosed, only to find that their feet kept getting larger. At some point in time, they ended up with an increase of a full size or more. I have occasionally seen increases of two-and-a-half sizes over a two-year period in adults!

This situation is especially a concern for kids, whose feet always seem to be growing. When in doubt, get new shoes. Too expensive? Don't be afraid to buy some of the inexpensive shoes on the market. The $9.95 models wear just as long as the fancy ones for $99.95. Unfortunately, once kids see enough shoe commercials on TV, they may only want the expensive brands.

Actually, children should go barefoot as much as possible. When shoes are necessary for children, find them the best-fitting, thinnest shoes with the least support. And that goes for grown-ups too — don't be afraid to spend as much time as possible barefoot. It not only helps to correct existing problems, but also prevents common foot problems seen in many older people.

# SELF-HEALTH MANAGEMENT

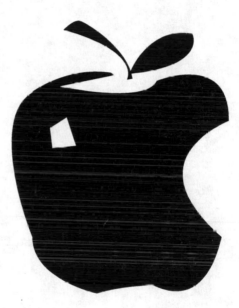

# 28 The Self-Health Revolution

Today there's a revolution afoot in the world of health care. Growing numbers of people are beginning to realize they must take responsibility for their own health. This revolution finds people shifting their efforts from crisis intervention to disease prevention. Instead of just regular visits to the doctor, these people are seeking information that can help them not only live longer but also enjoy a higher quality of life. Disease is not an unavoidable option for these people. The prospect of spending 12 completely dysfunctional years at the end of a lifetime is just not acceptable to them. In fact many people now rank longevity and quality of life as their No. 1 goal, and also recognize the enormously important role that diet, nutrition and exercise play in reaching this goal. I call this revolutionary movement *self-health management*.

In addition to longevity and quality-of-life issues, many people also are fed up with the expense of the modern health-care system. Health care is the single largest sector in the United States economy, consuming approximately $1.6 trillion annually. Health costs are projected to rise 6.5 percent per year in this decade, growing to 16 percent of gross domestic product in 2010 from about 13.5 percent at present. This projected growth is being fueled by factors including technological advances in the health-care industry and an aging population that will require the use of more and more health-care resources on a per capita basis.

Along with this, the Census Bureau projects that the proportion of the population age 65 and over — the age group with the highest health costs per person — will rise to 16.5 percent in 2020 from about 12.5 percent today. Baby boomers that today make up approximately 28 percent of the U.S. population will represent 67 percent of all those over 50 in America by 2010, posing a profound challenge to the entire health-care system.

As the patient base grows, an ever-expanding array of medical technology, devices and drugs enables these patients to undergo more tests and diagnostic procedures, take more drugs, see more specialists and be subjected to increasingly aggressive treatments. The advances in medical technology have increased the life expectancies of an increasingly large number of medically complex patients, many of whom require a high degree of monitoring and specialized care as well as rehabilitative therapy.

With the costs and demands upon the system skyrocketing, even the health-care industry has begun to realize that the only option is to shift the focus to preventing diseases rather than treating them. The medical establishment has long kept preventive medicine on the back burner, instead focusing on diagnosis and treatment of disease. However, within the last 15 to 20 years, concerned segments of the medical community began a massive effort to explore preventive measures.

The cornerstone to promoting health, maintaining wellness and preventing illness is information that empowers individuals to assume personal responsibility for healthy diet and lifestyle practices, and the self-discipline to incorporate these practices into daily living. In this regard, more effort is being made to boost individual responsibility, including incentives by employers and insurers for patients who exercise, eat the proper foods, lose weight and stop smoking. Many in the medical profession are now advocating that more funds be put into health education so that less money will be needed to treat various diseases that can be prevented. If health care is not addressed by these methods, chronic illnesses such as diabetes, arthritis, heart disease and cancer will affect a growing percentage of the population, and health-care costs will continue to escalate.

Despite this trend in the health-care system, the overwhelming evidence of the revolution toward self-health management is the increasing recognition and acceptance by the general public of the effects of diet, nutrition and lifestyle on achieving and maintaining optimal health and human performance.

**A Word about Weight Loss and Disease**
Statistics on the number of Americans who are overfat or obese are staggering, and change all the time. Unfortunately, instead of decreasing, these numbers seem to be swelling, right along with average waist sizes. Even recent television commercials and sitcoms have begun to feature overfat individuals as characters, a sad commentary on our increasingly overweight society. Also unfortunately, the condition of being overfat or obese is a contributing risk factor for almost every disease known to mankind, including heart disease, cancer and diabetes.

If you are overfat or obese it is crucial that you get this condition under control before it seriously affects your health. Many of the principles promoted in this book — diet, nutrition, aerobic exercise and stress control — also are principles that promote healthy weight loss and proper weight maintenance. Some major principles in particular that help with weight management are:

- Limit your carbohydrate intake to amounts your body can tolerate and eliminate refined carbohydrates and sugars.

- Include proper amounts of protein, healthy fats, vegetables, salads and fruit as part of a balanced diet.

- Rev up your metabolism by increasing the number of smaller meals you consume throughout the day.

- Improve your fat-burning system through easy aerobic exercise.

By following these guidelines as well as others presented throughout this book, you should reach and maintain your optimal weight without following faddish diet plans that in the long term usually only result in extra weight gain.

### Outlasting Rather than Conquering Disease

Many experts point out that there is a maximum biological limit to aging. By shifting health-care strategy toward ongoing prevention rather than last-minute intervention, we seek to defer the onset of degenerative diseases to a point beyond the maximum age limit.

For example, an individual who is on a course of degeneration leading toward the onset of cancer at age 60 may be treated with therapies designed to delay the onset to age 130. If that person dies naturally at age 110, the onset of the cancer will have been avoided. This is "outlasting" disease. The result is a phenomenon called "squaring the survival curve," a concept promoted by James Fries of Stanford University, who says: ". . . many people with the early stages (of disease) never progress to the later stages during their lifetimes."

Delaying the course of what is known as the universal degenerative process means an individual need not expect a life of slow declines and failing capacities — as they often saw with their parents and grandparents. Instead, robust health can be maintained into old age. The bottom-line benefits? Better, cheaper and user-friendly health care. The National Science Foundation agrees: "Postponing universal decline would lower, strikingly, per-capita costs for older persons, starting with the 45 to 49 cohort. Chronic costs would be delayed and their duration reduced. Individuals would tend to stay healthy longer and decline more abruptly."

All this sounds great, but is it more than just philosophy? Let's look at a hypothetical example of a person who is born relatively healthy, then falls into a long period of dysfunction with subtle but growing symptoms, ending in a disease state. We'll choose a person with carbohydrate intolerance, following the current health-care model.

Some babies begin life with stress. Our future patient may have been adversely affected by being fed formula or sugar water shortly after birth, or by excess maternal stress. This stress, coupled with genetic programming (perhaps a grandparent was diabetic), may predispose the baby to develop a less-stable blood-sugar mechanism, adversely affecting the nervous system.

Within the first three years of life the baby's nervous, hormonal, immune and digestive systems develop significantly. Also during this time, psychological makeup is developed. The nervous system, at any stage of development, is especially vulnerable to periods of low blood sugar, sure to occur in this young person. During the early years of life, a number of unhealthy patterns and physiological imbalances may be formed.

By age 12, this carbohydrate-intolerant teenager begins to develop symptoms. These include behavioral problems, various types of "learning disabilities," allergies, and asthma. Some girls even develop menstrual problems. As time goes on, intestinal symptoms and fatigue set in, and blood sugar may remain unstable. Some experts have linked blood-sugar problems to drug use and criminal activity. If brought to the attention of a mainstream medical doctor, he or she would probably rule out disease, and conclude that the problem may be psychological. Perhaps counseling would be recommended.

Before reaching age 20, this person attempts to lose weight through dieting. This vacillates from starving to lowering fat intake, accompanied by increased consumption of carbohydrates. It begins the process of yo-yo dieting, in which a lower caloric intake decreases metabolism, which results in some short-term weight loss, with the final consequence of weight gain.

To this point, this person would probably not have sought traditional health care for these seemingly minor but annoying problems. Over-the-counter drugs and other remedies provide symptomatic relief; effective marketing strategies promise help is just a pill away.

By the second through third decade of life, the carbohydrate-intolerant person usually becomes a patient. And at this point, many of the symptoms have worsened: fatigue, intestinal bloating and decreased concentration. Addictions are common — to sweets, caffeine, alcohol, tobacco or other drugs.

Many symptoms are now observable and measurable. Dizziness caused by a significant blood-pressure drop upon standing is common. Blood pressure may begin to elevate. Abnormal glucose-tolerance tests are sometimes found, but more often appear normal. Other signs include increased fat stores, seen in the abdomen in males, and the buttocks and face in females. Blood fats, especially triglycerides but also cholesterol, may begin to increase. More common and diffi-cult to measure early is a clogging of the arteries with fat.

If seen by a traditional doctor, the patient may be put on a diet to help relieve the symptoms. This diet may be high in carbohydrates, and low in fat, red meat, eggs and cheese. And the symptoms just get worse.

Exercise is sometimes recommended. But with no direction, the patient frequently exercises too intensely in the hope of burning more calories. This leaves this patient worse off, usually with a more pronounced aerobic deficiency.

Soon after this stage, around the fifth decade of life, measurable patho-logical, or disease states appear. They may include high blood pressure, high blood fats (triglycerides and/or cholesterol) and problems handling blood sugar. These signs may now be accompanied by named diseases: hypertension, hyper-lipoproteinemia and diabetes. There is now a very high risk for coronary artery disease, and if fat accumulates, blocking the flow of blood to the heart, bypass surgery may be the only way to prevent death. In many patients, all of these end-result diseases appear. At this stage, conservative measures such as exercise, diet and nutrition require more stringency to be effective, but still can play a major role in therapy. If disease is too advanced, more extreme countermeasures may be needed, such as surgery.

The last stage of life, the so-called golden years of the 60s and up, can literally be quite painful for both patient and family, and a great expense for all, including society. Our patient, now a medicated, hypertensive, overweight diabet-ic on the verge of requiring bypass surgery, remains at high risk until the end. But modern medicine has helped lengthen the life span. When death comes, it comes not only with pain and suffering, but also with great expense.

Could this scenario be changed? Could the suffering and expense be pre-vented? Clearly the answer is yes. And it's not just a philosophy; we can see it in action in people who follow the right path towards health and fitness.

### Treating Functional Illness

Recognition of functional illness early in life, when it's more easily and inexpen-sively treated with conservative measures, including lifestyle changes, makes the most sense. This is the true meaning of prevention. In medicine, prevention is thought of as a screening process, such as "screening for cancer" to find it early when it's more treatable. I prefer to think of prevention as postponing that can-cer and not allowing it to progress during your lifetime.

There's another important issue here: Waiting for medical intervention at this later stage may save and prolong your life, but too often the resulting quali-

## Finding a Health-Care Professional

The concept of self-health management is fairly straightforward: You manage your own health. But sometimes along life's journey you need advice or treatment. This is when finding a good health-care professional may be helpful.

Good health-care professionals are in great demand because there are too few of them. The first thing to do when seeking a health-care professional is to ask around. Mention to your friends or relatives that you're looking for a certain type of health-care professional. This may be a nutritionist, massage therapist, meridian therapist (acupuncturist), chiropractor, medical doctor or perhaps an applied kinesiologist.

Once you have a name you can find out more by talking with current patients or clients. Find out what they like and dislike about the professional they see. The important questions include those about how much time is spent on typical visits, if questions were adequately answered, and if the professional took the time to treat the person as an individual rather than a number. Also seek out information about philosophical compatibility — you don't want to work with someone who is opposed to how you have chosen to live your life.

Before making an appointment, don't be afraid to call a professional's office for information about how he or she practices. This is not unlike an interview: You want to know about someone before developing a professional relationship.

Once you make an appointment, take note of how this practitioner addresses your needs and concerns. If you have a good feeling about your visit, plan another as necessary. But if you don't feel comfortable, whether you can explain it or not, search for another health professional. It may take some time to find a person that's best for you.

The biggest problem in our current health-care system is that by going to see a particular health-care professional, you're most likely only going to get that person's specialty as treatment. For example, if you visit an acupuncturist, you'll get acupuncture; visit a surgeon, you often get surgery; visit a dietician, you'll get diet advice. But what if you have both surgical and nutritional needs for the same problem? It's uncommon to find a practitioner who can address all your needs, or who will refer you to another specialist, although these health-care professionals do exist and are worth seeking out. This is why you must actively manage the entire process. It's up to you to find the best health-care practitioners that match your needs.

ty of that life is unacceptable. Witness the many nursing home elderly who are not sure where they are, and do not recognize their families. Or even 60- and 70-year-olds, living alone or with family, but unable to enjoy a full and active life. These folks may have a decade or more of living left, but it may be a decade of pain and frustration and great expense.

Currently in the United States, it's accepted that people spend an average of 12 years of dysfunction at the end of their life spans, unable to care for themselves and just waiting to die, often slowly, in pain and confusion.

These problems can and are being addressed, but on such a small scale hardly anyone notices. There are those in their 70s who are active on a daily basis, people in their 80s who regularly play tennis and golf and go for a walk every day, and those over 100 who are functional human beings. These are people who, for the most part, have followed the basic rules and are reaping the benefits. They will die with dignity, typically during a good night's sleep.

We are not fated to live and die with a game plan we don't control. We can alter the quality of our lives, and influence the quality of our children's lives.

In this section about self-health management I discuss many topics regarding dysfunction and disease and how you can take a proactive approach to true prevention. By effectively managing your own health you may not only be able to avoid disease, but also limit your exposure to the health-care system, attain greater quality of life and reach the finish line of your life journey in good health rather than in dysfunction. The most powerful tool you have in this quest is information and that is what I have tried to provide here. The only thing left for you to do is embody this information by applying it to your own self-health management strategy.

# 29 Brain Power

It's estimated that one in four people in the United States suffers from some form of mental or emotional disorder, and many more have diminished brain function. Human error, a common result of diminished brain function, is the cause of the majority of automobile and airplane accidents, as well as other costly mistakes. Similarly, lack of memory represents the serious failure of an important brain function. In most cases these problems are preventable through proper diet, nutrition and lifestyle.

Do you remember where you were when President Kennedy was assassinated? Maybe you hadn't been born yet. How about when the space shuttle *Challenger* exploded? Or when the World Trade Center collapsed? Most people have vivid memories of where they were when these intense events occurred.

The vivid memory associated with these types of events has to do with optimal brain function. It's an example of how powerful an influence the blood-sugar mechanism can be on the brain. The reason people can remember intense events so clearly is that the adrenal-response mechanism triggers optimal levels of blood sugar, shown in studies to enable the brain to record and remember associated events, names, faces or other factors even years and decades later. A variety of influences, from diet, nutrition, exercise and stress, can also affect blood-sugar. Some are helpful for brain function, but in many cases, these influences result in poor brain power. It's possible to mimic this ideal brain function with good dietary, nutritional and lifestyle habits.

## Blood Sugar and Your Brain

Learning, memory, and all other cognitive function have an undeniable relationship with stable blood sugar. Whether you're healthy, without existing blood-sugar problems, or are aware of some type of problem you already have, blood-sugar irregularities can hit you at any time, adversely affecting brain function.

While many clinicians and patients have struggled to define the problem, many years of ridicule by the medical establishment kept this issue from being researched adequately. But the research is now underway and a number of studies are showing up in medical journals. These publications were once highly critical of any discussion of blood-sugar problems, except for rare instances, or in the case of diabetes.

The brain and its unlimited capability are highly dependent upon a delicate balance of blood sugar. If the level of blood sugar rises too much, or falls too low, the brain has an immediate reduced capacity. This means you don't remember as well, don't respond as well to external stimuli, and can't learn as easily. Reductions in overall mental performance can follow.

We're all too familiar with reduced mental capacity. From early in life a child's poor learning can be a problem. As adults we joke about "brain damage." In older adults cognitive dysfunction such as Alzheimer's disease is on the rise. Creativity, in both children and adults, is another mental process that can be compromised when blood sugar is not balanced.

Blood sugar is controlled by a number of factors. Diet, nutrition, exercise, and a variety of lifestyle factors such as stress all play crucial roles.

Brain chemistry is very dependent upon the balance of carbohydrate and protein in the diet. High-glycemic carbohydrates, especially sugar and processed flour products, can reduce and impair brain function due to the effects of insulin as discussed in chapter 6. The application of this fact is simple: Don't go to work or send your kids to school after a breakfast of high-glycemic cereal or other sweets. Virtually all breakfast cereals have a very high glycemic index. Most adults know not to drink and drive, but many still go to work, operate vehicles or embark on other activities that require optimal brain function without the right fuel. A better choice would be an egg-based breakfast without sweets or fruit juice. Blood sugar can be controlled exceptionally well by snacking on healthy items. Eating five or six meals daily, rather than the two or three most people consume, will help stabilize blood sugar, allowing the brain to do its job properly.

Vitamins, minerals and essential fats are also vital for brain function. Perhaps the most important nutrients, especially for youngsters, are the omega-3 fats EPA and DHA, as discussed in more detail later in this chapter. Most children won't get enough from food, so supplementation is often necessary. The omega-3 fats are key ingredients for growth and development of the brain and eyes.

Arachidonic acid contained in animal foods is another essential fatty acid necessary for brain function. Other nutrients include the B vitamins, iron and a number of minerals including magnesium. Foods such as beef and a variety of vegetables can supply these nutrients.

Stress, and hormones produced in excess due to stress, can wreak havoc on blood sugar and reduce brain function, as discussed in the next chapter.

Physical activity can help improve brain function in many ways. Exercise can help improve blood-sugar regulation, stress control and other factors. Too little, or too much exercise can impair brain function. So seek a balance.

## Ritalin Works Just Like Cocaine

For more than 40 years, it was not known how the popular drug Ritalin — prescribed to millions of children with Attention Deficit Hyperactivity Disorder (ADHD) — really worked. But scientists have recently found that Ritalin acts just like cocaine by chemically manipulating the brain's dopamine system to reduce distraction and increase attention signaling.

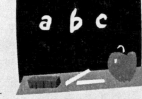

Ritalin was one of the first in what would become a group of drugs used to treat ADHD and related behavioral problems. Today Ritalin and similar drugs are used by up to six million children. Many adults also take the drug, along with untold numbers of illicit users.

Like cocaine, Ritalin is classified as a Schedule II controlled substance by the Drug Enforcement Administration. It is among the most addictive and abused drugs that are still legal.

Despite its widespread use, Ritalin does not address the cause of the problem, but merely offers symptomatic effect. The side effects of Ritalin are numerous and include decreased appetite, which can adversely affect the child's nutritional state, as well as retarded growth, insomnia, increased irritability and rebound hyperactivity when the drug wears off.

In addition, while ADHD is often associated with brain chemistry, it is important to note that ADHD and similar behavioral problems often have other contributing factors, including psychological dynamics and social stress.

Psychotropic drugs have a reported effectiveness rate of about 75 percent. However, the effectiveness of natural remedies that include the use of dietary supplements and diet modification is also reported in scientific studies to be about 75 percent.

Children diagnosed with ADHD have been found to have low levels of omega-3 fats in their cells. Omega-3 fatty acids are key components in the brain and are central to neurological function and visual acuity. Studies show low omega-3 levels correlate with poor behavior scores and teacher scores of academic abilities.

This is due not only to lack of omega-3 fats in the diet, but may also be the result of having trans fats in the diet, which could displace omega-3 fats in cells. Trans fats come from hydrogenated and partially hydrogenated oils found in many food products, especially junk food. In addition, excess intake of omega-6 fats from common vegetable oils can result in low omega-3 levels in the body.

Since most children don't eat foods containing omega-3 fats, taking an omega-3 dietary supplement may be essential.

### Brain Pain

When we consider mental energy, it's clear thinking and creativity we want, rather than that foggy feeling or depression. When you have a thought or feel a sensation from the outside world, it's the result of major chemical reactions in your brain. Billions of messages are sent throughout the brain and the nerves on a regular basis by brain chemicals called neurotransmitters. Different neurotransmitters make you feel different ways: high, low, sleepy, awake, happy and sad. Sometimes the brain may have too many of one type of neurotransmitter or not enough of another. As a result, you may feel too high or low, or too sleepy. A common end-result symptom may be depression or anxiety. When these problems develop, antidepressant drugs are sometimes prescribed to manipulate brain chemistry, in hope of balancing neurotransmitters and relieving symptoms.

For most people, diet can have a profound effect on brain chemistry, often as much effect as drugs. What you eat, or don't eat, for dinner can influence your sleep, your dreams, and how you feel upon waking. And what you eat, or don't eat, for breakfast can determine your human performance for the day.

Most of the 40 or more types of neurotransmitters are made from amino acids derived from the protein in your diet. Certain vitamins and minerals are also required for their production, including vitamin B6, folic acid, niacin, iron and vitamin C. There are many important neurotransmitters related to mental function. They include serotonin and norepinephrine — the two most commonly discussed substances. Let's look at how a traditional meal affects most brains, and why the confusion surrounding this issue continues.

### Turkey Day Syndrome

Most people think getting sleepy after Thanksgiving dinner is due to the turkey — more specifically, the tryptophan content of the turkey that can sedate the brain. Tryptophan, an amino acid that can produce a sleepy feeling when given in high amounts, is relatively high in turkey. But while this notion is promoted year after year in the media, it's completely false.

The reason so many people get sleepy after Thanksgiving dinner is something I call TDS — Turkey Day Syndrome. It's not caused by eating turkey, but rather by eating all the trimmings. It's the same as sleepiness produced by any other meal high in carbohydrates. In the case of a typical holiday meal, it's the bread, potatoes (including sweetened sweet potatoes), gravy (made with flour), cranberries (sweetened with sugar), and of course those extra servings of pie (there's always more than one type to taste). Throw in some alcohol and it's no wonder you're craving more than just one pot of coffee.

While turkey does have a high amount of tryptophan, it has many other amino acids that prevent tryptophan levels from elevating in the blood (thereby not affecting the brain). The foods that affect the brain most in your Thanksgiving meal are the carbohydrates. They cause a rise in a brain neurotransmitter, serotonin, which has a calming, relaxing, sedating effect. And the more sugar and starch you eat, the more sedating its action.

Sleepiness after any meal may be indicative of carbohydrate intolerance. So if you often feel this way, it's time to evaluate, or re-evaluate your eating habits.

Any high-carbohydrate meal, such as pasta, or a meal containing lots of sweets, causes the brain to produce more serotonin. This also increases insulin production, which raises the amount of tryptophan entering the brain, which then produces still more serotonin. The individual who is easily agitated or mentally overactive may benefit from a carbohydrate meal. Too many carbohydrates, however, can produce too much serotonin in many people, causing oversedation or even depression. If you're a student, executive, or just want to use your brain, you might find that eating sufficient carbohydrate to adversely affect brain chemistry is counterproductive.

While sweets are traditionally thought of as providing energy, they are in actuality mentally sedating. Sometimes sweets may give the feeling of a pick-up, but that is very short-lived, until insulin lowers the blood sugar, resulting in more fatigue.

Processed carbohydrates (white-flour products, sugar, most cereals and breads) and potatoes will have a quicker and more adverse effect on brain chemistry than whole, unrefined carbohydrates (whole-grain bread, brown rice and oatmeal). These whole foods contain natural fiber and natural fats which slow the conversion to glucose. Fruit juice, though natural, is also void of fiber and is very concentrated. The glucose is quickly absorbed with the same potentially negative effects on brain chemistry as regular sugar.

If you need a mental pick-up, try eating some protein. A protein-based meal with little or no carbohydrates causes your body to produce less insulin, and provides a higher amount of tyrosine and increased norepinephrine levels. This neurotransmitter has a stimulating effect on the brain. The person who needs a mental pick-up or who gets sleepy after a meal could benefit from eating a high-protein meal with little or no carbohydrate.

Drugs are sometimes used to balance brain chemistry. Depressed patients are given medication to restore balance to the neurotransmitters. Prozac, Elavil, Aventyl, Tofranil and Norparmin are antidepressants that affect the balance of serotonin and norepinephrine. (Tranquilizers, such as Valium and Ativan, have a different function and affect other neurotransmitters.) But these medications have side effects, including reductions in glutathione, the most important and most powerful antioxidant which protects the brain from chemical damage.

If your brain chemistry isn't balanced, you may benefit by simply altering your diet. Consider these recommendations:

- When going to an important morning meeting, lecture, class or exam, don't eat a carbohydrate breakfast such as cereal or pancakes. Especially avoid the orange juice, doughnut and so-called "energy" bars that are high in sugar. A carbohydrate meal may upset your brain chemistry and make you less alert. Instead, have a high-protein, low-carbohydrate breakfast: eggs, cheese or meat with one piece of whole-grain toast and no potatoes. Drink vegetable juice (V-8, tomato or carrot) instead of fruit juice.

- If it's a long, important day, you'll want to do the same thing at snack time and at lunch. Avoid high-carbohydrate snacks such as candy, rolls and other common break-time foods. Eat cheese, nuts or other protein foods instead.

- If you're having more than one day of important activities, make dinner a meal with carbohydrates to help you relax and sleep during the night. Just be careful not to consume carbohydrates beyond your tolerance level. The next morning, start your day again with a high-protein, low-carbohydrate meal.

### Omega-3 Fats and Brain Function

While proper essential-fatty-acid balance is important for many systems of the body, it is also necessary for proper brain function. Imbalances in essential fatty acids — particularly deficiencies in omega-3 fats — have been implicated in depressive disorders in adults and behavioral problems in children and adolescents, including Attention Deficit Hyperactivity Disorder, difficulties with learning, impulsivity, hyperactivity, aggression and anger.

Researchers at the National Institutes of Health have identified positive effects of omega-3 fats on the brain and also established a direct link between an imbalance in fatty acids and depressive disorders. In fact, it appears that omega-3 fats affect neurotransmitters in ways that mimic the effect of some antidepressant medications. These fats coat the brain-cell membrane, serving a protective function when neurotransmitters are fired in the synaptic phase.

Omega-3 fats have other benefits in brain function as well. Fish oil may help moderate release of the stress hormone cortisol, resulting in improved brain function. Additionally, omega-3 oils have been found to reduce the severity of degenerative brain diseases that lead to memory loss and dementia, while omega-3 deficiency has been implicated in Alzheimer's disease. Also, a lack of adequate levels of docosahexanoic acid (DHA), a fatty acid found in fish oil, has been implicated in depression, with inadequate amounts affecting the degree of severity.

## Other Brain Requirements

The brain's 200 billion cells also have numerous nutritional requirements for good function. These include a number of vitamins and minerals, and most importantly, water. Any dietary inadequacy can potentially have a dramatic impact on brain function. Numerous neurological symptoms have been associated with a deficient diet, including aggression, learning disabilities, depression, hyperactivity and memory problems.

There is an important relationship between folate levels and depression. Numerous studies show that many people with depression also have low levels of folate. Consuming foods containing this nutrient can significantly improve depression in these people. For this reason, anyone considering antidepressant medication should first be screened for folate levels through a blood test for homocysteine, the best indicator of folate levels in the body. For depressed individuals who have low folate levels, adequate folate intake and utilization may be as effective as Prozac or other antidepressant drugs for treating mild, moderate and severe depression. Folate is contained in green, leafy vegetables and fruits; in some cases, fruit, especially citrus, can be a better source than leafy vegetables. Synthetic folate, or folic acid, from most supplements may not be as effective or as well utilized in many people as folate obtained from real food sources.

Sodium, potassium, magnesium and calcium are also important for sending messages through the brain. Iodine has an important role in brain maturation, beginning in the fetus soon after conception. In children, a strong association has been made between iron deficiency and Attention Deficit Hyperactivity Disorder. Zinc is important for growth and maturation of the brain and is used for many chemical reactions in the brain, especially those related to behavior. Copper is also related to growth and maturation of the brain. This doesn't mean that just taking these nutrients will automatically improve brain function. In fact, just taking a lot of nutrients can have the opposite effect.

**Herbal Relief for Depression**

Clinical trials have repeatedly found St. John's Wort as effective as prescription antidepressant drugs for treating mild to moderate depression. In addition, this herb has fewer and less-dangerous side effects. While the chemical action of St. John's Wort is not fully understood, many scientists believe the combination of antioxidant polyphenols and flavonoids, especially hypericin and pseudohypericin, may function synergistically to regulate neurotransmitters in a fashion similar to antidepressant drugs.

Those products that are standardized for consistent dosage are best, as many St. John's Wort products have varying levels of active ingredients. St. John's Wort also contains many other beneficial nutrients, including essential oils, glycosides, resins, tannins and rutin. Many of these substances also can be found in other health-promoting foods such as vegetables, green tea and cocoa.

Side effects include possible interactions with oral contraceptives, medications for AIDS and cholesterol-lowering drugs. Always check with your health-care professional before taking St. John's Wort, especially if you are on any prescription medication.

While copper deficiency has been associated with deterioration of mental function and physical coordination, too much of this mineral can have the same results. Manganese, like copper, is both important for proper brain function and has potential for adversely affecting the brain if taken in excess. Lead and mercury are both toxic to the brain and pose real health problems throughout the world. Lead poisoning has been known for centuries. For years scientific literature has described mercury poisoning, ranging from contamination of fish through accumulated methyl mercury (introduced to the food chain by industrial waste) to consumption of grain treated with mercury fungicide. The debate over dental fillings is still a concern to many in the scientific community.

Vitamin B6 is another important brain nutrient, and is used in the regulation of certain neurotransmitters. Because estrogen can reduce the levels of vitamin B6, this may be important for some women, especially those taking birth-control pills and on estrogen-replacement therapy.

Though caffeine isn't considered a nutrient, it is a drug. This is obvious to those who regularly consume caffeine in coffee, and to a lesser degree in tea, cola and chocolate. The most obvious effect is increased mental performance and alertness, though negative brain effects appear after a couple of hours, when the drug wears off and you crave more. The physical side effects can also be unhealthy. Some people can tolerate, without harmful effects, a certain amount of caffeine each day. Others shouldn't take any. It's up to you to determine if your body can tolerate caffeine, and if so, how much.

As you can see, a variety of dietary and nutritional factors can help improve brain power — beginning at fetal development and continuing throughout your life and into old age. Both children and adults can improve their brain function by choosing foods that match their needs. For example, eating a balanced ratio of protein, unrefined carbohydrate and fat can help optimize blood sugar, thereby improving cognition, learning and memory. Certain dietary supplements can also be very helpful, especially quality fish-oil products. Making dietary choices that ensure proper nutrient intake, such as adequate folate levels, can also be helpful in regulating brain function and improving conditions such as depression. In addition to these dietary considerations, another factor that can improve brain function is proper management of stress levels, the topic of the next chapter.

# 30 Simplifying Stress

Stress is such an incredibly powerful influence that even if you are doing every-thing right in terms of diet, nutrition and exercise, it can still crush your efforts to stay healthy. Prolonged periods of too much stress can contribute significantly and directly to many conditions, ranging from reduced quality of life to deadly diseases such as cancer, heart disease, Alzheimer's and many others. Between these extremes, stress influences most pre-disease or sub-clinical illnesses, including fatigue, bacterial and viral infections, inflammatory illness, blood-sugar problems, weight gain, intestinal distress, headaches and most other physical problems. Stress-related problems account for more than 75 percent of all visits to primary-care physicians and are responsible each day for 1 million people needing to take time off work. So stress comes with a monetary price tag as well as a toll on your health. In this chapter I'll explain what stress is and what you can do about it when it's out of balance.

Coping with stress can become such a complex problem, it in itself can become part of the stress you accumulate in life's journey. It's important to remember that stress is a normal part of life and health, and excess stress is not without a remedy. The body has a great coping mechanism — the adrenal glands. However, when this system is overworked, problems can result.

We can do many things to help ourselves, but first we have to under-stand what stress is. While stress is a complex subject, we can simplify it by say-ing there are three main types of stress: physical, chemical and mental/emotion-al. These types of stress can have many different effects. Moreover, each individ-ual responds differently to various combinations of types of stress.

## Physical Stress

Physical stresses are strains on the physical body. Overworking a muscle or mus-cles is an example of a physical stress. Slight physical stress is what makes exer-cise beneficial, and is an example of how some stress can help promote health. However, too much physical stress without adequate recovery can potentially result in many problems. Another physical stress is wearing shoes that don't fit right; while you don't always feel it in your feet, it may cause problems elsewhere in your body. Likewise, dental problems can affect more than your mouth. Other physical stresses include poor posture, eye strain, and many other situations that adversely impact the physical body. Physical stress can result in physical problems, but also in chemical or mental/emotional problems.

### Chemical Stress

Chemicals from any source can affect body chemistry and cause stress. Chemical stresses include dietary and nutritional imbalances such as too much or too little food or nutrients, excess caffeine or drugs, and ingestion of chemicals from food and water supplies. Other sources of chemical stress include those in the air — second-hand smoke, indoor and outdoor air pollution and many others. Chemical stresses can cause indigestion, fatigue, insomnia, or even physical and mental/emotional problems.

### Mental and Emotional Stress

Mental and emotional stress is the type with which most people are familiar. This includes tension, anxiety and depression. Setting unrealistic goals, or none at all, can also be stressful. Mental stress may contribute to pain, moods of anxiety or depression, and loss of enthusiasm or motivation, and can lead to physical and chemical problems as well. Mental stress also affects cognition, including sensation, perception, learning, concept formation and decision-making.

### Stress, Good and Bad

Stress can be defined as any factor that affects the body or mind, causing the body to react and adapt. This process is managed, to a large extent, by the adrenal glands, located on top of each kidney. These small glands are also responsible for physical, chemical and mental recovery from a typical day's activity, which is one type of stress. Adapting to stress takes time and energy, and the more stress you experience, the more time and energy it takes to adapt.

Stress can come from anywhere: your job, family, other people, your emotions, infections, allergic reactions, physical trauma and exertion, even the weather. Remember, not all stress is negative. Since it evokes a reaction in the body, the outcome may be a positive one — the benefit of exercise is one example. By mildly stressing your body, over time and through adaptation, your body performs better. But that same stressor — your workout — can become negative if you go too far beyond the body's ability to recover from it.

Usually people are stressed in more than one area, frequently by all three types. Stress is cumulative. The response to a physical stress from the weekend's yard work may be amplified by Monday's chemical stress of too much coffee and food that isn't nutritious, further compounded with a family-related mental stress on Tuesday and another with the boss on Wednesday. All of this will affect your performance at an important meeting on Friday.

The weather is also a potential stressor, with certain people more vulnerable. Weather stress may affect us physically, chemically or mentally. Extremes in temperature or humidity, very low barometric pressure, and the sun are stressors. Seasonal Affective Disorder (SAD) is a good example of how the weather at certain times of year (typically in the fall and winter) can have a dramatic effect on many people.

Some people have a greater ability to tolerate stress. A small part of this coping mechanism of the adrenal glands may be genetic. Those without *me.* strong adrenals still have an option: stress control.

## Making Your Stress List

In addition to helping your body adapt better to stress, cutting down on stress is an obvious remedy. Being more aware of your physical, chemical and mental stress factors is a requirement for improving health. The key to controlling stress is to first carefully assess it, with the goal of diminishing or eliminating some of your stress. Reducing or eliminating stress factors is easier if you write them down on paper.

On a page, make three columns, one each for physical, chemical and mental stresses. In each category, write down your stresses. This may take several days to complete since you probably won't think of all your different stresses right away. When you're done, prioritize by placing the biggest stress of each category on top. Then, work on reducing or eliminating one stress at a time. Or, if you can handle it, work on one stress at a time from each category. Reducing or eliminating unnecessary stress from your life will give your body a better chance to cope with other stresses you may not be able to change right now.

As you make your list put a star by the stresses over which you have some control. This may include unhealthy eating habits like rushing or skipping your meals, drinking too much coffee or not taking time to exercise.

Simply draw a line through those stresses that you can't control. If there's nothing you can do about them anyway, don't worry about them. Take them out of your mind. Many people expend lots of energy on stresses they can't or won't do anything about. This may include job stress or the weather, though in reality, almost any stress can be modified or eliminated — it's just a question of how far you're willing to go to be healthier and more fit. As time goes on, you may want to reconsider some of the items you've crossed off. You'll realize that

**235**

changing jobs is a must, or moving to a more compatible climate is necessary for your health.

Once you can "see" your stress listed on paper, it will be easier to manage. Start with your starred stresses first, because you have control over them — not that it's always easy. Circle the three biggest stresses from the starred list and begin to work on them. You may be able to improve on some and totally eliminate others. Some will require habit changes. It's a big task, but one that will return great benefits. When you've succeeded in eliminating or modifying each one, cross it off your list and circle the three next most stressful ones, so you always have three to work on.

You're probably familiar with other strategies for dealing with stress, though you may not use them. Here's a reminder:

- Learn to say "no" when asked to do something you really don't want to do. Ask yourself if you really want to do this.

- Decide not to waste your time worrying about the past or the future. That's not to say you should ignore the past or not plan for the future.

- Learn some relaxation techniques, and perform them regularly. An easy walk by yourself can be a great meditation, along with the physical benefits. Yoga or other meditative activities are helpful for some people.

- When you're concerned about something, talk it over with someone you trust.

- Simplify your life. Start by eliminating trivia. Ask yourself: "Is this really important?"

- Prioritize your busy schedule; do the most important things first. But don't neglect the enjoyable things. Before getting out of bed in the morning, ask yourself: "What fun things do I have planned for today?"

What's most important about stress is that too much of it interferes with rest. Or more accurately, recovering from excess stress requires more rest. If you don't get enough rest, usually in the form of sleep, your health and fitness can be adversely affected. One of the questions to ask yourself is whether you're getting enough sleep, considering the amount of stress you have. As you will see, one of the symptoms of excess stress is insomnia.

### Case History

*Dave had numerous complaints — physical, chemical and mental. A Wall Street executive, he was building a new home and had spring and fall allergies that nearly incapacitated him each year. Dave spent more than two weeks making and pondering his stress list. After discussing all the issues with family and friends, he decided to make some changes. Dave and his family sold their partially built house, moved to a nicer climate, and he secured a job with less stress. Though the pay was less, so were the taxes and other stresses. Within six months, Dave felt 15 years younger. Even his family was healthier, and they felt closer.*

A common mental stress is obsession. I'm not talking about compulsive disorders or extreme problems, but the common obsessions many of us harbor. Too often, these "mental fixations" become irrational when it comes to important things such as exercise and diet. For example, go to a typical health club and what do you see: mirrors. People want to see what they look like on the outside, often not thinking about what they're doing to their insides. Or how about your diet habits? Are you obsessed with calories and grams of fat? I had a patient who avoided eating broccoli because it contains fat — the natural fats found in the flowers!

Another trademark of obsession is found in the compulsive exerciser who fears that taking a day off will ruin all that was gained. The fact is, resting can improve fitness. Counting miles is another common obsession among runners. At the end of your training week you tally up 38 miles; so you run two extra just to get to 40, despite feeling tired. Or you jog the 80 meters from your car to the office twice daily and include that in your weekly mileage. All these obsessions are significant stresses and can adversely affect your health and fitness.

By learning to take control of the various types of stress in your life, you can improve the quality of your life, reduce the risk of dysfunction and disease, and also help your adrenal glands regulate stress. Maintaining proper adrenal function is central to good health and fitness, and is the subject of the following chapter.

# 31 Adrenal Function

Charles Darwin said it's not the fittest who survive, nor the most intelligent, but those who can best adapt to their environment. Today, we refer to this adaptation as coping. No matter what type of stress you encounter during your life journey — be it physical, chemical or mental/emotional — your body has an efficient system for coping. It's called the adrenal system and it is regulated by a small gland on top of each kidney. In addition to the adrenal glands themselves, the sympathetic nervous system plays a vital role in coping with stress and can be considered a vital part of the adrenal system. The adrenal glands not only are essential for stress coping and optimal human performance, but also for life itself. The adrenals produce a variety of hormones that control many bodily functions, including stress regulation, sex and reproduction, growth, aging, cellular repair, electrolyte balance and blood-sugar control.

Cortisol is a key adrenal hormone associated with stress. When your body is under high stress, cortisol will be elevated. In chronic stress states, and poor coping, cortisol levels will either be too high or too low. Cortisol has an important relationship with blood-sugar regulation and fat-burning — two functions that may be adversely affected when cortisol levels are not normal.

The sex hormones, including estrogens, progesterone and testosterone, are adrenal hormones that help both males and females maintain proper sexual function and reproductive health. The adrenals also make dehydroepiandrosterone, or DHEA (mostly in the form of DHEAS), which is the precursor to the estrogens, and testosterone.

Both epinephrine and norepinephrine are two other key hormones that help regulate the metabolism and play vital roles in the body's reaction to stress.

Since stress is regulated by the adrenal glands, high levels keep your adrenals quite busy. But problems can arise when the stress hormones become imbalanced. For example, too much cortisol suppresses the immune system, lowering the body's defense mechanism, making it more susceptible to colds, flu and other viral and bacterial infections. Chronic high cortisol can also impair memory and contribute to Alzheimer's disease.

## The General Adaptation Syndrome
Our knowledge about stress and adrenal function began in the early 1900s, when famous stress-research pioneer Hans Selye began to piece together the common

triad of signs resulting from excess adrenal stress. They include adrenal-gland enlargement, depressed immunity and intestinal dysfunction. Selye eventually showed how the adrenals react when confronted with excess stress. This *General Adaptation Syndrome* has three distinct stages.

The first stage begins with the alarm reaction, in which there is an increase in adrenal hormone production. This is an attempt by the adrenals to battle the increased stress. If it is successful, adrenal function returns to normal. During this stage, a variety of mild symptoms may occur: spotty tiredness during the day, mild allergies or even some nagging back, knee or foot pain. If, over time, the adrenals fail to meet the needs of the body to combat the stress, they enter the second stage, called the resistance stage.

During this period, the adrenal glands themselves get larger, a process called hypertrophy. Since the increased hormone production of the first stage couldn't counter the stress, the glands enlarge in an attempt to do the same. During this stage, more advanced symptoms may occur, including fatigue, insomnia and more serious back, knee or foot pain. If the stress is still not controlled, the adrenals enter the third stage, called exhaustion.

The exhaustion stage is just that: extreme tiredness. The adrenal glands are unable to adapt to stress. At this point, the person usually becomes seriously ill, physically, chemically or mentally.

**Are You 'Stressed Out'?**
How many times have you heard someone say, "I'm stressed out"? Well, the comment may be accurate. Excess adrenal stress — or an insufficient adrenal response to adapt to stress — is a common problem. It is often the result of chronically overstimulated adrenal glands. This can be due to stress from work, rearing children, or many other sources. It's sometimes due to poor diet, financial problems or family stress, or a combination of several stresses. Overexercising — either too much duration or intensity — is also a common cause of excess adrenal stress. The cause of the excess adrenal stress, or the reason the glands are not able to counter existing stress, must be found and corrected. If you are successful, the body's natural powers are released and often health and fitness will improve dramatically. *Please Vary*.

I should be clear that we aren't talking about adrenal disease, rather, the gray area between normal adrenal function and disease.

Ten common symptoms of adrenal dysfunction are listed below. Check off any that pertain to you. They can be caused by other imbalances in the body. But taken together, they make up the most common symptoms of adrenal dysfunction.

☐ **Low energy.** This is common especially in the afternoon, but could happen anytime, or all the time. The fatigue can be physical, mental or both. When the adrenals are too stressed, the body uses more sugar for energy, but can't access fat very well for energy use. This can significantly limit your energy.

☐ **Dizziness upon standing.** Standing up from a seated or lying position can make you dizzy. This is because not enough blood is getting to the head quickly enough. Check your blood pressure while lying down, and then immediately after you stand. If you suffer from adrenal dysfunction, you will notice the systolic blood pressure (the first number) doesn't rise normally, though it should be higher when you're standing by about 6 to 8 mm.

☐ **Eyes sensitive to bright light.** Adrenal stress often causes light sensitivity in your eyes. You may need to wear sunglasses or have difficulty with night driving because of the oncoming headlights. You may even misinterpret this as having bad night vision. Some people find their nearsightedness (ability to see distances) improves after improving adrenal function.

☐ **Asthma and allergies.** Whether you call it exercise-induced asthma, food allergies or seasonal allergies, it's the symptom and not the cause. Other people could be exposed to the same allergens without getting symptoms, so the cause is not the allergen, it's poor adrenal function.

☐ **Musculoskeletal symptoms.** Problems in the low back, knee, foot and ankle are often caused by adrenal problems. These areas can become mechanically unstable and produce symptoms such as low-back pain, sciatica and excess pronation in the foot, leading to foot and ankle problems.

☐ **Stress-related syndromes.** The problems referred to as burnout, overtraining (overexercising) and nervous breakdown are almost always the result of adrenal exhaustion. While occasionally these problems become serious enough to warrant medication or hospitalization, adrenal dysfunction occurs long before this point.

☐ **Blood-sugar-handling stress.** For years, many people, including doctors, talked about low blood sugar. It's difficult to measure and obtain accurate indicators of this elusive problem, in part because it's usually secondary to adrenal dysfunction. Without proper adrenal function, one common result is the inability of the body to control blood sugar. Symptoms include constantly feeling hungry, being irritable before meals or if meals are delayed, and having strong cravings for sweets and/or caffeine.

☐ **Insomnia.** This is a very common adrenal problem. Many people with adrenal dysfunction fall asleep easily (often because of exhaustion) but wake in the middle of the night with difficulty getting back to sleep. This may be due to high levels of cortisol, which during sleeping hours should be low. Many people say they wake up in the night to urinate. But it's usually the adrenal problem that awakens them, and then they get the urge to urinate.

☐ **Diminished sexual drive.** This is a common symptom of adrenal dysfunction. Adults who have lost their sexual desire are usually low in the hormone DHEA, which makes estrogen and testosterone. Eventually, this can also adversely affect the strength of bones and muscles.

☐ **Seasonal Affective Disorder (SAD).** This is common, especially in the fall and winter. As the hours of daylight lessen and the temperature drops, many people go into a mild state of hibernation. The metabolism slows, and the body and mind become sluggish, sometimes resulting in a mild or moderate depression. In my experience with patients, this often corresponds with adrenal dysfunction. Contributing to this dilemma may be a combination of stresses: the weather, lack of sunlight and even the start of the holiday season. People don't eat as well as they intend, are less active, and weight gain is common.

Recognizing these 10 common symptoms of adrenal dysfunction can be useful in your self-assessment. You may also want to test some of your adrenal-hormone levels with the help of a professional. The best test for adrenal hormones measures cortisol and DHEA, and is performed over the course of a full day and evening, rather than just a single test. Saliva samples are collected at 8 a.m., noon, 4 p.m. and midnight. Sometimes a single blood test is done to measure these hormones, but since adrenal hormones normally fluctuate throughout the day, if a sample is taken at 9 a.m., for example, you know only the levels at that time. It's possible that at 9 a.m. the hormone levels are normal but at 4 p.m. they are very low. As for blood tests, going to a hospital or doctor's office sometimes causes additional stress, which can interfere with an accurate result.

With an awareness of the signs and symptoms of adrenal stress, you can make some appropriate lifestyle changes to improve adrenal function and possibly solve many of your problems. Earlier I discussed the importance of making your stress list. Now, let's look at some of the other factors related to improving adrenal function: diet, nutrition and food extracts, exercise and lifestyle.

## Diet and Adrenal Stress

One of the most important dietary factors related to adrenal stress is the consumption of refined sugar, not just sugar in desserts and the table variety added to coffee and cereal, but hidden sugars in many foods. Products including ketchup, mayonnaise, bread, crackers and canned food contain sugar, sometimes in large amounts.

If you have any adrenal dysfunction, eliminate sugar. Until you get your adrenals working better, desserts, candy, sweet snack foods, sugared drinks, and sugar in coffee or tea must be avoided. (After your adrenals function better, small amounts of sugar are usually tolerated.) As discussed throughout this book, consuming sugar quickly raises the blood-sugar level, causing the hormone insulin to be released, which then lowers blood sugar. Either or both of these reactions can be a stress requiring compensation by the adrenal glands.

Excess consumption of other refined carbohydrate foods such as bread, rolls, pasta, cereals, white rice and even potatoes, milk and fruit juice, can also create adrenal stress. How much is too much? Perform the Two-Week Test if you're not sure.

Caffeine is also a common source of adrenal stimulation, and it's addictive. Coffee, tea and colas are the main sources. If you have a functional adrenal problem, assess your caffeine intake. For many, no caffeine is best. For others, a cup or two of coffee or tea may be tolerable. You must determine, as objectively as possible by listening to your body, how much caffeine your body can tolerate.

Always eat breakfast. Avoid too much carbohydrate (nearly all cereals are refined and have hidden sugars) and be sure to include some protein with your breakfast; eggs can be the cornerstone of an ideal breakfast.

People with adrenal stress often need to snack between the three main meals, even every two hours in the early stages of recovery. Healthy snacking habits were discussed in chapter 19. In general, low-carbohydrate snacks are best; cheese, nuts, vegetables and hard-boiled eggs are some good options. Avoid sugars, refined starches and fruit juice.

**Nutrients and Food Extracts for Adrenal Stress**

A person with adrenal dysfunction may be in need of many different types of nutritional support, ranging from certain micronutrients and dietary factors intended to improve nutrient absorption, to substances intended to spark production or replace certain hormones. Since the hormonal system is very complex, it's recommended that you seek the input of a health-care professional to correct a hormonal imbalance. In general, those with adrenal dysfunction may require one or more of these micronutrients: vitamins B2, B6, C or pantothenic acid.

For many types of adrenal stress, especially those that cause insomnia, zinc may be useful. Studies show this important mineral can help lower high cortisol levels that accompany adrenal stress. Taken right before bed, for example, zinc may improve sleep patterns.

Choline is another nutrient commonly needed by some people with adrenal stress, in part due to the relationship of choline with the nervous system. Individuals who are always on the go, overworked and trying to do too much are examples of those who may benefit from choline. Small amounts several times a day may be very helpful. The best source of choline in the diet is egg yolks.

Intestinal dysfunction almost always accompanies adrenal stress, which may or may not be noticed as a symptom. With increased stress, intestinal efficiency diminishes, including the ability to absorb nutrients from your diet. L-glutamine is an amino acid used by parts of the small intestine to help improve nutrient absorption during times of stress, and while you're on the road to improving adrenal function.

There are a variety of adrenal products available in the marketplace, including those made from bovine adrenal sources. These supplements may have great value for the person who has adrenal dysfunction. But care must be taken to match the right supplement with the specific need. This is an area in which a competent health professional can be helpful.

**Exercise Considerations**

Exercise can both help and worsen adrenal dysfunction, depending on the type of activity you perform. In general, easy aerobic activity is helpful for all except the person in the end stage of adrenal exhaustion. In this case rest may be most important until adrenal function is improved. More intense anaerobic workouts usually worsen adrenal problems at any stage.

- If you do not already exercise, a 20- to 30-minute easy walk, five times per week, is a great adrenal therapy.

- If you already work out, consider replacing some of your exercise with easy aerobic exercise, such as walking. It will build the small aerobic muscle fibers, promoting more fat-burning and increasing circulation, both of which will help adrenal function.

- Stop all anaerobic workouts, including weight-lifting and any exercise that raises the heart rate above your aerobic level. Once adrenal function is improved, anaerobic exercise can be resumed, though the balance of aerobic and anaerobic exercise must be maintained.

### Other Lifestyle Factors

One of the most therapeutic things you can do to reduce stress is get a massage. Licensed massage therapists perform various types of massage, and you and your therapist should determine which best suits your needs. If you haven't had massage therapy, start with Swedish massage, which can help reduce adrenal stress.

Sunlight on the skin and through the eyes is important to proper adrenal function and can help improve dysfunction. Do not stare directly into the sun; just spending time outdoors provides sufficient photo stimulation through the skin and eyes. Natural, full-spectrum light from the sun can help the brain regulate adrenal hormones, especially at times of the year when daylight is lessened. This is because the messages from the brain to the adrenal glands are affected by light. Window glass (home, office and in your car) and prescription and non-prescription glasses and contact lenses can filter out the stimulating part of the light spectrum. If you normally are exposed to little or no sun, take a walk during your lunch break to get some natural light (even on a cloudy day). For indoor use, consider replacing your regular light bulbs and tubes in locations where you spend considerable time with full spectrum lights. This will mimic the light you aren't getting from the outdoors.

Evaluate your sleeping habits. Are you getting at least seven hours each night? If not, you may need more. Adrenal stress increases the need for recovery. Decide what changes are needed to ensure that you are getting enough sleep.

*music*

Research shows that music pleasant to the adrenal-stressed listener can lower high cortisol levels. Play music while in your car, at work or at home. Choose music you like. The radio can have stressful commercials and commentary. Play the music you liked during the more stress-free and happiest times of your life.

*meditation*

Various meditation methods can counter stress. Walking or listening to music can also be meditative. Find what works for you, what takes your mind off your stress, makes you dream and gets you away from it all each day. Don't forget you still have to work on your stress — just some other time. These options, along with your stress list, can help you deal with your stress in effective ways.

**Other Natural Hormones**

Hormones play a major role in your physical, chemical and mental well-being. The key to optimal hormonal performance is balance. To create this balance, a number of lifestyle factors must be considered. The most important factor is stress. Too much or too little stress can have devastating effects on hormonal balance. Two important hormones, produced by both men and women, that have drawn much attention in recent years are estrogen and progesterone. As you age, and with increased stress, the production of these hormones is diminished. This occurs when cortisol rises, diminishing the production of DHEA, and subsequently, diminishing estrogen, testosterone and progesterone. Replacing these natural hormones with synthetic versions has been a topic of major controversy. What most don't realize is that natural alternatives are available.

**Estrogen**

This most well known of hormones is actually a group of about 20 compounds. The most important estrogens are estrone, estradiol and estriol. The different estrogens have unique roles in the body. For example, estradiol is the most stimulating to the breast, and is the estrogen related to increased risk of breast cancer. Estriol protects against breast cancer. When both are produced by the body, you have the right balance. A variety of benefits are attributed to the effects of natural estrogens, including prevention of hot flashes, better memory and concentration, slowing of the aging process, and reduced depression and anxiety.

Synthetic estradiol (Premarin) is the estrogen that places you at high risk for breast cancer. This is due to the fact that it's not broken down in the liver as quickly as your own natural estrogens (affecting the cells for a longer time). Premarin, made from the urine of pregnant horses, simply doesn't function exactly like the estrogens made in the human body. In addition to natural estradiol, other natural estrogens have synthetic companions and are marketed under various brand names.

One of the common risks of taking synthetic estrogen is dosage. The most common symptom of too much estrogen in your system is water retention. This leads to breast tenderness and swelling, weight gain and headaches. Excess estrogen can also lower blood sugar and increase your cravings for sweets. Too much estrogen also increases your risk of uterine cancer and gall-bladder disease.

While estrogen is often "sold" to patients by touting the benefits of building strong bones, estrogen doesn't actually do this. It will decrease the rate of bone loss that occurs naturally throughout life. Progesterone and testosterone are the hormones that have the greatest impact on the growth of new bone — something your body is also always promoting.

**Progesterone and Testosterone**

Unlike estrogen, which is a group of hormones, progesterone is the only hormone in its class. Progesterone has many functions in the body. It increases sex drive, improves sleep, builds bone mass, protects against breast and uterine cancer, improves carbohydrate tolerance, helps burn fat, prevents water retention, and in many people it has a calming effect on the nervous system.

Provera is a synthetic version of progesterone, one that is given to many women. However, it doesn't have the same functions as the natural hormone. While natural progesterone acts like a diuretic, Provera makes you retain salt and water, and can make you gain body fat. Too much of this synthetic hormone can cause bloating, depression, fatigue, increased hair on the body and increased weight gain. Provera can also cause your body to diminish its own production of natural progesterone, forcing you to rely more on outside sources. Other synthetics can cause birth defects, epilepsy, asthma and heart problems.

It's important to note that both estrogen and progesterone work together. In a real sense, they balance each other when in their natural state.

Testosterone is also a naturally occurring hormone made by both men and women. This hormone increases muscle mass, healing and bone building, increases sex drive and energy, and is a very important hormone for other areas of the metabolism. The synthetic version is methyltestosterone.

**Getting Yours Naturally**

The ideal scenario is to have your body make the types and amounts of hormones necessary for you. That amount varies from day to day and year to year (even from minute to minute). If you interfere with this delicate mechanism, imbalances can occur. Some people produce too little hormone. If this happens, taking synthetic hormones sometimes is a guessing game with potential side effects much worse than the signs and symptoms for which they were prescribed. Unfortunately, millions of people take unnatural hormones without knowing there are natural alternatives.

One real option to synthetic hormone therapy is to use natural plant hormones. Many plants contain natural hormones, but the most common are soy products, peanuts and yams. Licorice root is also high in natural hormones.

Food extracts of natural hormones are available for those who require a concentrated amount. For instance, estriol is a natural estrogen available by prescription from a pharmacy. (For more information, and a list of doctors who prescribe estriol, call the Women's International Pharmacy, 800-279-5708.)

For those who need natural progesterone, a non-prescription product called Pro-Gest is available in a cream that can be absorbed through the skin rather than taken by mouth (your liver breaks down much of the natural hormone taken orally). For those who require both natural estrogen and progesterone, a product called OstaDerm cream can be very helpful. Micronized natural hormone supplements are absorbed in the mouth and are also effective.

Wild yam extracts are also available in health-food stores. These are a relatively mild form of natural progesterone. But beware of the many natural hormone products on the market; there are now dozens. Most are very low in natural hormones, and some hardly have any.

For menopause, premenstrual syndrome, or other hormone-related imbalances, the use of natural hormones can improve your quality of life. What's most important is to understand that no one has to live with the pain, displeasure and discomfort that too many doctors have told patients are normal with aging.

### Case History

*Sally was in her early 40s and had a variety of hormone-related symptoms, including hot flashes, insomnia and body-fat increase, all beginning over the previous two years. Her doctor wanted her to start taking synthetic hormones, but she was uneasy since her family history included breast cancer. My first choice was to try to get Sally's adrenal function improved, as tests showed her cortisol and DHEA levels to be far from normal. After several months of making lifestyle changes, Sally's symptoms improved by about 50 percent. At this time, I recommended she begin using a natural progesterone cream, once per day after showering. Within three months, Sally began feeling better, and within six months, felt more like she did when she was 30.*

# 32 Chronic Inflammation: The Hidden Epidemic

Inflammation is typically thought of as swelling, pain or discomfort, perhaps in your joints, sinuses or intestines. But for many people chronic inflammation occurs without symptoms and may be the cause of other health problems. A full spectrum of disorders are associated with chronic inflammation — from severe functional problems such as fatigue, hormonal imbalance and reduced immunity, to serious diseases such as osteoporosis, heart disease and cancer. In fact, chronic inflammation is now considered to be a major risk for coronary heart disease.

Most people don't know that chronic inflammation can lead to dysfunction and serious disease. Likewise, many are unaware that inflammation is, in fact, a normal bodily function. Acute inflammation is a healthy action when all systems are working properly. Without it, you would not recover from a day at the office, a walk to the mailbox, or a workout, and even a small splinter in your finger could worsen and possibly result in death.

There are three important functions of acute inflammation. One is the first step in the healing or repair process after some physical or chemical injury or stress, no matter how minor. Inflammation also prevents the spread of damaged cells that could cause secondary problems in other areas of the body. A local infection, for example, can be contained due to the inflammatory response, instead of causing a bodywide infection. Inflammation also rids the body of damaged and dead cells.

Acute inflammation is caused by various trauma such as a fall, or microtrauma from repetitive day-to-day activity, such as a workout or even something as simple and seemingly benign as typing. It is also caused by intense exercise such as weight-lifting and competition, infections, toxins, birth-control pills and stress.

Normally, the inflammatory cycle is almost like an "on-off" switch. Inflammation is turned on by inflammatory chemicals when needed for healing and repair, then turned off by anti-inflammatory chemicals when not needed. It's when these anti-inflammatory chemicals are not present in sufficient quantity, or there's too much inflammatory-causing stress, that the switch stays on. The outcome is chronic inflammation.

Chronic inflammation has other causes as well. For instance, increased body fat, including larger waist sizes, produces inflammation bodywide. More than

60 percent of the U.S. population over the age of 17 years is overweight, and as many as one in six may be obese. Children also are not immune to chronic inflammation, especially if they are overfat.

The results of inflammation include those all-too-familiar injuries — chronic "itis" conditions such as tendinitis, faciitis and arthritis. Chronic inflammation could also ultimately lead to disease or ill health, including cancer, heart disease, Alzheimer's and others, as discussed later in this chapter.

### Two Faces of Inflammation

As you can see, inflammation can best be viewed as two separate conditions. *Acute inflammation* is the body's normal initial response to a physical or chemical stress that requires healing and repair. This form of inflammation is typically accompanied by pain, swelling, redness and heat. A closer look at an area of inflammation reveals that the small blood vessels are dilated, bringing in more blood, as well as other fluid, causing warmth and swelling of the area. The acute inflammatory response to a typical physical or chemical stress can last up to three days, with the entire repair process taking up to six weeks.

*Chronic inflammation*, on the other hand, is an ongoing abnormal condition that can cause or is associated with ill health and disease. It's only when acute inflammation does not, or cannot, complete its task, that chronic inflammation results. This distinction is emphasized because many people think of inflammation as something to eliminate, typically through drugs or through the use of popular supplements. The transition from acute to chronic inflammation may take place due to continued physical or chemical stress, such as smoking or ongoing infection. More often it's due to biochemical influences such as an imbalance of dietary fats, an absence of specific substances that adversely affect the anti-inflammatory production, and/or specific nutrient problems.

It's possible to work with inflammation to improve its natural course of action. This involves learning how to help your body heal itself, and correct and prevent a course that could lead to ill health and disease. But first you must have a handle on just how well your inflammation system is working.

### Assessing Inflammation

For some people, the presence of inflammation is obvious. But most people with chronic inflammation are not aware of it because the signs and symptoms may not be apparent. Therefore, some type of evaluation is important. The following survey may help guide you in determining your potential for inflammation. Check the items that pertain to you:

☐ Do you eat restaurant, take-out or prepared food daily?

☐ Do you consume milk, butter or cheese regularly?

☐ Do you consume corn, soy, safflower or peanut oils regularly?

☐ Do you consume margarine regularly?

☐ Do you consume products that contain hydrogenated or partially hydrogenated oils regularly?

☐ Is your diet low in fresh wild salmon, sardines, and flaxseed oil?

☐ Do you have a history of atherosclerosis, stroke or heart disease?

☐ Do you have a history of osteoporosis?

☐ Do you have a history of ulcer or cancer?

☐ Do you have a history of inflammation ("itis" conditions) such as arthritis, colitis, tendinitis, etc.?

☐ Do you have allergies, asthma or recurring infections?

☐ Do you have chronic fatigue?

☐ Do you have increased body fat?

☐ Do you perform weekly anaerobic exercise, such as weight-lifting, hard training or competition?

☐ Do you perform regular repetitive activity (jogging, cycling, walking, typing, etc.)?

Even if you check only one or two of the above items, it indicates an increased chance of having chronic inflammation. This can be confirmed with blood tests performed by your doctor. The following are common blood tests used for the assessment of inflammation.

### Tests to Determine Inflammation

The C-reactive protein (CRP) blood test is the most accurate screen for inflammation and can detect very low levels. The normal range should be 0.0 to 1.5mg/dl (or 0.00 to 0.15 mg/L). This test can also predict future risk of coronary heart disease and stroke even in otherwise healthy individuals. The best suggestion is to have a CRP performed yearly, when other blood tests are ordered. If the result is not normal, retest every three to six months to monitor the effectiveness of any program you use to reduce inflammation, such as the suggestions that follow.

Other tests include the erythrocyte sedimentation rate (ESR). This common blood test for inflammation can be performed when blood is taken for other tests, or with a finger prick. Compare your results to the normal range given by the lab. A complete blood count measures white blood cells and may also indicate inflammation. Compare your results to the normal range given by the lab.

Body temperature is a general indicator of inflammation. However, it is not the best test as only more significant inflammation will elevate temperature. The normal temperature is 98.6° F, with only a very slight range of normal (a few tenths of a degree); morning and nighttime readings are the lowest and late-afternoon temperatures the highest.

### Causes of Inflammation

As I have discussed, many things can cause inflammation. Following is a list of common contributors.

- Trauma, such as an injury received in a fall, is a common cause of significant inflammation.

- Microtrauma, which includes such subtle actions as walking, typing and any repetitive motion, normally produces inflammation.

- Intense physical activity, such as anaerobic exercise — including high-intensity training, weight-lifting and competition — also causes significant inflammation.

- Chemical stresses such as food allergies, hay fever, handling or breathing harsh chemicals (cleaners, gasoline, cosmetics and toiletries, etc.), air pollution and others can cause inflammation.

- Infections from bacteria, virus, fungus or yeast also cause inflammation.

- Increased body fat can cause inflammation because fat cells pro-duce inflammatory chemicals such as cytokines and series 2 eicosanoids. This is especially serious in those who are obese.

- Birth-control pills and hormone-replacement drugs may promote chronic inflammation. Women who take estrogens have higher levels of C-reactive protein, indicating increased chronic inflam-mation. Naturally high levels of estrogens in women may not have the same inflammatory effect since these levels are still much lower than those from drug hormone therapy.

As discussed below, nutritional imbalances can cause chronic inflamma-tion. This is especially true with dietary fats — herein lies the key to controlling inflammation from a dietary standpoint.

**Diet and Inflammation**
Many of the chemicals involved in both inflammation and anti-inflammation are heavily influenced by your diet. This was discussed in chapter 11 and is reviewed here because of its importance. The four items below can have a dramatic effect on reducing unwanted inflammation.

- Balance your intake of dietary fats as discussed in chapter 11. If you have a fat imbalance that affects your inflammatory system it may be necessary to supplement your diet with essential fats. For most people this means omega-3 supplementation. I formulated Nature's Dose™ Infla-min Anti-Inflammatory Complex specifically for people who need to reduce inflammation, but this supplement also has other powerful health benefits as well.

- Eat foods that combat inflammation. As discussed later, these foods include citrus peel, ginger, raw sesame-seed oil, turmeric and garlic.

- Make sure you have all the nutrients necessary for maintaining bal-anced fats, including vitamins B6, E, C, and niacin and the minerals magnesium and zinc.

- Avoid specific foods and lifestyle factors that disturb the balance of fats, discussed as follows.

In addition to balancing fats and getting the right nutrients to make anti-inflammatory chemicals and prevent excess inflammation, other dietary factors can have a significant effect on your inflammation-control system.

One of the worst habits for those with inflammation is the consumption of trans fats. These include hydrogenated and partially hydrogenated oils. These fats block the production of anti-inflammatory chemicals. The most common foods containing these fats are margarine and shortening. In many cases, hydrogenated fats are listed on labels. But in some cases, they're not. For example, most peanut butters, or items containing peanut butter, contain hydrogenated fat even though it may not be listed as an ingredient. Ingredients listed as "natural peanut butter" do not contain these bad fats, but an ingredient listed as just "peanut butter" usually does contain them.

Consuming high amounts of carbohydrate in your diet can also lead to reduced anti-inflammatory chemicals, and excess inflammation. Carbohydrates include sugar and sugar-containing foods, such as sweets and other desserts. Also, pasta, bread, cereal, potatoes, rice, syrups, fruit juice and foods with hidden sugars (ketchup, most peanut butter and many other foods) are very high in carbohydrates. If you want to reduce your inflammation, it's vital to moderate your carbohydrate intake. This is accomplished in part by significantly reducing your sugar intake, and relying mostly on unrefined carbohydrates such as fruits, berries, brown rice, legumes, etc. Reductions in dietary-carbohydrate intake typically accompany increased protein consumption, which is also important for producing anti-inflammatory chemicals.

Ginger is a powerful food that can combat inflammation. This light-brown root, available in most grocery stores, can be used raw in many foods and is sometimes pickled — a common item in Japanese restaurants. Ginger can be used in salads, or to make tea, or is added to many dishes for its pungent flavor. Developing a habit of using ginger regularly in your meals can be very helpful in controlling inflammation. Its therapeutic effects are so powerful that if you don't like its taste, or don't eat it often, taking ginger in supplements should be part of your anti-inflammatory efforts. Turmeric, a spice that's in the ginger family, also has anti-inflammatory properties. Many people have it on their shelves but use it infrequently. It's commonly used as a natural coloring agent, and is a major ingredient in curry powder.

Many people eat citrus fruit but toss the peel. They are throwing out some of the most important nutritional factors. The oil in citrus peel contains limonene, a powerful phytonutrient. One way to eat the peel is to drop the entire fruit into a blender or food processor and then eat or drink the resulting "slush."

Or, eat the skin, or at least the white parts, when eating the fruit. This is more enjoyable when the fruit is tree-ripened, which makes for a much sweeter skin.

Foods in the onion family can help reduce inflammation, especially garlic and onions. In our culture, garlic and onions are often avoided due to the odor after eating them. But both have great therapeutic benefits and should be part of your daily diet, even if it's just in your evening meal. Other foods in the onion family include shallots and chives.

Inflammation is also produced from free radicals — chemicals produced in the body from oxidative stress. This reaction is much like the rusting of metal. Free radicals themselves contribute to ill health and disease. Rancid fats, chemicals in your food, water and air, and other chemicals from cleaners, cosmetics and even your car, promote free-radical production. Certain high-dose supplements, such as iron and copper, can also produce dangerous free radicals. The body uses antioxidants to eliminate free radicals, obtaining most through the diet in the form of certain vitamins, minerals and phytonutrients. Fresh vegetables are the best source of antioxidants and phytonutrients. If you're not eating five, six or more servings of fresh vegetables daily, consider taking a real-food antioxidant supplement that has phytonutrients. Free radicals are discussed in more detail in chapter 35.

### Fighting Inflammation with Lifestyle
An important lifestyle factor that contributes to inflammation is excess stress of any type. This can be in its physical, chemical, or mental/emotional forms. As discussed in chapters 30 and 31, excess stress overproduces certain hormones that impair the production of anti-inflammatory hormones. In addition, the hormones testosterone and thyroxin in higher-than-normal levels can also interfere with anti-inflammatory chemical production. Other items that can promote inflammation include excess alcohol, which would be a chemical stress. While moderate amounts of wine can provide some very important phytonutrients and help reduce inflammation, large amounts of any alcoholic beverage, especially the sweet ones, should be avoided.

### Functional Illness
If you have chronic inflammation and allow it to continue unchecked, a full spectrum of functional problems, such as fatigue, hormonal imbalance and reduced immunity may result. Fatigue may be among the more common results of chronic inflammation. Other problems associated with chronic inflammation include:

☐ **Lowered immunity.** This can result in frequent infections, including colds and flu, and yeast and fungal infections such as Candida. Asthma, allergies and other problems may also be due to low immunity and chronic inflammation.

☐ **Hormonal imbalance.** This can include many aspects of the hormonal system, especially the adrenal stress hormones, reducing your ability to cope with stress. Sex hormones — estrogen, progesterone and testosterone — can also be adversely affected, resulting in diminished sex drive and reproductive function. Reduced thyroid function can also result due to inhibition of thyroid-stimulating hormone.

☐ **Nervous-system imbalance.** This includes increased activity of the sympathetic nervous system, potentially leading to increased tension, rising blood pressure, disturbed blood sugar, anxiety or depression, or other problems.

☐ **Digestive distress.** Among the problems that can result are poor digestion, gas formation, heartburn and various inflammatory conditions such as colitis and ileitis. Poor absorption of nutrients can be another result, creating an entire series of potential problems throughout the body.

☐ **Chronic pain.** Inflammation produces pain-stimulating chemicals throughout the body. This results in a reduced pain threshold.

☐ **Cataracts.** Another common condition that develops with age is cataracts, and inflammation seems to play a major role in the development of this eye disease. Chronic inflammation has been shown to predispose healthy individuals to future risk of age-related cataracts.

☐ **Gingivitis and periodontal disease.** These oral conditions are also associated with inflammation, and may be a silent cause of chronic bodywide inflammation.

☐ **Hair loss.** Loss of hair may be associated with inflammation in the scalp, specifically the hair follicles.

## Chronic Diseases

Chronic inflammation has been linked to more-serious diseases. It is now considered a major risk factor for cardiovascular disease. A variety of other disease states may be an end result of chronic inflammation, including ulcers and cancer, atherosclerosis, stroke, osteoporosis and even type 2 diabetes.

Other common diseases associated with inflammation have "itis" at the ends of their names: arthritis (inflammation of the joints), colitis (inflammation of the colon), tendinitis (inflammation of a tendon), etc. The inflammation may exist only in the early stages, such as with tendinitis, or become part of the chronic condition. Increased inflammation is also associated with chronic fatigue syndrome, and in studies, administration of inflammatory chemicals resulted in symptoms including anorexia and fatigue. It's possible that research will find other cause-and-effect relationships with chronic inflammation.

## Tendonopathy, Not Tendinitis

The musculoskeletal condition possibly most misunderstood by both patients and health-care professionals is tendinitis. Whether in the Achilles tendon, elbow or other areas where tendons can be abused or injured, by the time these problems are realized, the so-called tendinitis is usually not an "itis" at all. Experts call this common tendon problem tendonopathy — a term that more adequately describes the problem.

Tendonopathy results when injured tendons do not recover from repetitive, overuse injuries, or from daily repetitive activity. In other words, tendonopathy is usually the result of a dysfunctional inflammation system. The end result of this disrepair and lack of recovery is physical damage to the tendon's tiny collagen fibers. At this point the problem becomes chronic, but inflammation is usually no longer the issue. The pain may not be from inflammation but from dysfunction of the tendon, or often a nearby joint, ligament or muscle. In many cases the pain can come from more than one source.

Since there is usually no inflammation present with tendonopathy, treatment using anti-inflammatory drugs is not warranted, and the use of analgesics or other pain-control remedies is merely for symptomatic treatment. Some people continue to use the afflicted tendon, usually with the help of drugs to reduce the associated pain. However, reducing pain often results in the person using, or abusing, the tendon once again. The many ads for pain relievers are very successful in selling products that are not therapeutic, and often result in an aggravation of the problem.

Allowing the tendon to heal is the key remedy. As with most conditions, the course is very individual. In many people, the muscles associated with the injured tendon may not be functioning correctly. Getting help from the right health-care professional to restore proper muscle function can be an important part of any therapy.

Prevention of these common tendon problems is the best approach. When starting an exercise program, or performing any work you're not used to, keep it short with adequate periods of recovery, and be sure to adequately warm up and cool down for any activity. Avoid overtraining or other overuse. In addition, be sure your body has adequate levels of EPA from omega-3 fats.

Getting a handle on your level of inflammation may mean making some changes in your diet, nutrition and lifestyle, or finding ways to reduce stress levels. Controlling your inflammation now is an important step forward for your health. Not only will it improve your quality of life now, it will also pay off bigger benefits later in life by warding off dangerous, life-threatening illnesses.

# 33 The Big Picture of Heart Disease

Heart disease is the number one cause of death in the United States, and despite the abundance of low-fat and low-cholesterol foods and diets, the numbers keep growing. Today many people are rightly confused as to what actually causes heart disease. This confusion is at least partly to blame for many cases that could otherwise have been avoided through proper diet and lifestyle practices.

One of the most misunderstood subjects related to heart disease is cholesterol. Many people think that total cholesterol is the best — or only — measure for heart-disease risk. In fact, total cholesterol is not a very good indicator of risk. Many people who die of heart disease have normal total cholesterol numbers, and many with high cholesterol never develop heart disease.

Another common misconception is that eating foods that contain cholesterol significantly raises levels in the blood. In truth, many studies have shown that eating cholesterol does not alone substantially increase blood-cholesterol levels. Moreover, some studies show that not eating cholesterol can prompt your body to make more — and that eating eggs can improve your cholesterol numbers! When assessing risk for heart disease, it's best to look at the big picture. Rather than looking at one small piece of the puzzle like total cholesterol, or worse yet, cholesterol consumption, it's better to consider all the various contributing factors. These include the following:

- Total cholesterol, including HDL and LDL, can be a contributing factor.

- Triglycerides in particular give a good indication of heart-disease risk since carbohydrate intolerance is another very significant factor.

- Chronic inflammation, as measured by a C-reactive protein test, is now considered by many experts to be a better indicator of heart-disease risk than total cholesterol.

- High homocysteine levels also can significantly increase the risk of heart disease. Elevated homocysteine reflects inadequate levels of certain nutrients including folic acid, and vitamins B6 and B12.

Other nutrients are important for optimal heart function, including vitamins B1 (thiamin) and B2 (riboflavin). In addition, certain lifestyle factors also put you at risk for heart disease. For instance, you probably know that smoking poses a serious risk for heart disease, but few people realize that inactivity puts you at almost as great a risk as smoking.

With the exception of lifestyle issues, all of these factors are easy to evaluate with simple blood tests. Unfortunately, most people may know their total cholesterol number, but don't know as much about other risks. Worse yet, too many health-care providers still do not normally test for all of these factors. Let's take a closer look at each of these four key factors.

### Cholesterol Explained

The most important thing to know about cholesterol is that cholesterol itself isn't "bad," but rather something to be kept in balance. It's also important to understand that most of the cholesterol in the bloodstream is actually made by the liver. If you eat more cholesterol, your body prompts the liver to make less of it. But if you take in less, your liver makes more. That's why many people on a low-cholesterol diet still have high blood-cholesterol levels.

Actually, all cells in the body — including those of the heart — make cholesterol everyday. That's because cholesterol is necessary for many essential processes. For example, the outer surfaces of cells contain cholesterol, which helps regulate which chemicals enter and exit. As discussed in chapter 31, cholesterol is also used to make many hormones, including sex hormones and those which control stress. Cholesterol is also a key component of the brain and nerve structure throughout the body.

While there is a correlation between higher total cholesterol numbers and incidences of heart attacks, today the newest guidelines for evaluating risk call for a complete blood-lipid profile, as I have recommended for years. A blood-lipid profile test measures total, HDL and LDL cholesterol, as well as triglycerides.

### The Good Cholesterol

HDL cholesterol — high-density lipoprotein — is called "good" cholesterol because it protects against disease by removing accumulated deposits of cholesterol and transporting them back to the liver for disposal. So higher HDL numbers are generally healthier. It's best if you can divide your total cholesterol figure by your HDL number and get a ratio below 4.0, which is about the average risk for heart disease. Aerobic exercise, monounsaturated fats, fish oil and moderate alcohol can increase HDL. Stress, too much anaerobic exercise, hydrogenated fats and excess consumption of saturated fats and carbohydrates lower it.

More importantly, the recommendation that people substitute polyunsaturated fats for saturated can be devastating for HDL levels. If the ratio of polyunsaturated fat to saturated fat exceeds 1.5, HDL levels usually diminish, raising your cardiac risk. If your A, B and C fats are balanced, as discussed in chapter 11, you avoid raising your ratio above 1.5. Due to the heavy marketing of polyunsaturated oils since the 1970s, American diets now contain twice the polyunsaturated oil compared to diets of the 1950s and 60s. In addition, body-fat samples today show that levels of linoleic acid (an A fat) are at twice what they were 40 years ago.

### The "Bad" Cholesterol

LDL cholesterol — low-density lipoprotein — is known as the "bad" cholesterol. A recent trend in preventative medicine is to stress lowering LDL using lifestyle changes and even drugs. But it's really not the LDL itself that causes the potential harm or risk. It's only when the LDL oxidizes that it deposits in your arteries. Oxidation of LDL results from free radicals, in much the same way that iron rusts. While lowering LDL levels can make less of it available for oxidation, antioxidants from fruits and vegetables, and the right dietary supplements made from whole foods, can help prevent oxidation. Many factors that raise HDL also lower LDL. Nuts, fiber and soy protein are other dietary factors known to lower LDL, which is best measured when blood is drawn after a 12-hour fast.

Excess dietary carbohydrates can also adversely affect LDL levels. This is due to excess triglycerides from carbohydrates (discussed later) producing more, smaller, dense LDL particles, which are even more likely to clog arteries.

In addition, a lower intake of dietary cholesterol is linked to an increase of these more dangerous LDL particles. And to make matters worse, these types of LDL particles are also associated with the inability to tolerate moderate to high levels of dietary carbohydrates (i.e., insulin resistance) even in relatively healthy individuals.

### Factors that Affect Cholesterol Ratios

One of the worst scenarios for your cholesterol is if the HDL is lowered and the LDL and total cholesterol are elevated. Hydrogenated and partially hydrogenated fats (trans fats) do this. And many experts now consider the intake of hydrogenated fat to be a risk factor for heart disease. So avoid margarine and products containing this dangerous substance.

**261**

Eating too much saturated fat can raise LDL and total cholesterol levels. The worst offenders are dairy foods such as butter, cream, cheese and milk. Red meat such as beef, while it does contain saturated fat, can actually improve cholesterol levels. This is partly because, just as in eggs, about half the fat in beef is monounsaturated. In addition, much of the saturated fat in beef is stearic acid, a fatty acid that won't raise cholesterol and may actually help reduce it. The fat in cocoa butter also contains high amounts of stearic acid.

Fiber and fiber-like substances are also an important factor in decreasing total cholesterol and improving total cholesterol/HDL ratios. Most people don't eat enough fiber, especially from fresh vegetables and fruits, as discussed in chapter 15. I often recommend that people eat at least one raw salad daily in addition to at least five servings of cooked vegetables and one or two servings of fresh fruit or berries. These foods provide natural phytosterols, which help reduce cholesterol, and may be the reason early humans, who ate very large amounts of saturated fat, may have been well protected.

### The Sun and Your Heart

Vitamin D, the "sunshine vitamin," has a strong correlation with reducing the risk of heart disease — perhaps by as much as 30 percent! Vitamin D is produced by the action of sunlight on cholesterol contained in the skin. It is essential for calcium absorption from the foods we eat. Vitamin D levels therefore reflect calcium utilization by the body, especially in the bones and other tissues. Poor calcium utilization may result in this mineral being deposited in the arteries — a condition called arteriosclerosis. So spending some time in the sun is actually a heart-healthy activity. In fact, studies show that women with osteoporosis, also related to vitamin D deficiency, are much more likely to have heart problems.

Studies also demonstrate that more-frequent eating lowers blood cholesterol, specifically LDL cholesterol. This includes eating healthy snacks as was discussed in chapter 19.

### Case History

*Fred had a long history of high blood cholesterol. His many blood tests revealed some interesting numbers. When first tested three years previous, his total cholesterol was 288, and his HDL was 52. That's a ratio of 5.5 — too high a risk factor. Fred tried lowering his dietary cholesterol for six months, then had his cholesterol tested again. This time, the total was very similar, 276, but the HDL diminished too much, down to 41. That drastically increased his risk to 6.7. His doctor recommended taking a cholesterol-lowering drug. Six months later, the tests showed his total cholesterol down to 213, along with his HDL, which decreased to 31. Now his risk was even higher, with a ratio of about 6.9. Fred was finally convinced to try another approach. After six months of easy aerobic exercise, lowering his carbohydrate intake and eating the right fats, including eggs, his blood test showed total cholesterol of 191, and HDL of 58, giving a much better ratio of 3.3. A year later, Fred's test was even a little better.*

## The Triglyceride Factor

Triglycerides are another important piece to the blood-fat puzzle. These are fats converted from carbohydrates you have eaten. Normally, 40 percent or more of carbohydrates are converted to fat and stored. Some of these triglycerides end up stored as plaque on your artery walls. Many people focus on eliminating saturated fat and are unaware that eating too many carbohydrates is also associated with a higher risk for heart disease. Triglycerides, like LDL cholesterol, must be measured in the fasting state. Levels ideally should be under 100 mg/dl, though 150 is considered normal by most labs. If your triglyceride level is above 100, there's a good chance you're carbohydrate intolerant and need to cut back on eating these types of foods, especially those made with refined flour and highly processed sugars. Those with very high triglycerides often will see a dramatic reduction, sometimes to normal, after a successful Two-Week Test.

## Inflammation and Heart Disease

As discussed in the previous chapter, many people do not know they have chronic inflammation, but it is very common. Chronic inflammation is now considered to be as important a risk factor for heart disease as high cholesterol. In addition to heart disease, it may also be an early indicator of cancer and other diseases. C-reactive protein (CRP) testing provides a measure of bodywide chronic inflammation. This evaluation should be part of any regular blood test. Confirm that your level is in the normal range. The culprit behind chronic inflammation in most people is unbalanced consumption of dietary fats. Most people consume too much saturated fat, omega-6 vegetable oils and hydrogenated oils, and not enough omega-3 and monounsaturated fats. The proper dietary adjustments, coupled with

### Cholesterol Drugs: Costs vs. Benefits

A study published in *Circulation*, the official journal of the American Heart Association, indicates that major cholesterol-lowering drugs, the so-called statins, actually reduce inflammation, which is now believed to be as important a risk factor for heart disease as cholesterol. But considering the potential side effects of these drugs, and their high cost, statins are an inefficient way to lower cardiac risk by reducing inflammation. The study found the popular drugs Pravachol, Zocor and Lipitor significantly reduced inflammation, thereby reducing the risk of heart attack and stroke.

However, the long list of these drugs' side effects include liver damage and problems with neurological, intestinal and muscular function, as well as many others. In addition, patients must take this medication for many years and avoid alcohol. These drugs are also contraindicated for children, nursing mothers and women of childbearing age.

The irony is that the anti-inflammatory actions of these drugs may be more important than lowering cholesterol. It's a lot less expensive and safer to use appropriate dietary and lifestyle adjustments in combination with omega-3 fat supplementation to reduce inflammation. Indeed, the American Heart Association recommends first using more conservative means before prescribing medication, including diet, nutrition and exercise.

omega-3 fish-oil or flaxseed-oil supplementation, can correct many inflammatory problems.

### Folate, B Vitamins, and Cardiac Risk

Levels of homocysteine that are above normal are also now considered a more serious risk factor for heart disease than high total cholesterol. High homocysteine levels indicate that your body has inadequate folic acid, along with vitamins B6 and B12. Not coincidentally, inadequate levels of these nutrients are also associated with brain dysfunction and possibly Alzheimer's disease. Consuming folic acid, B6 and B12 through your diet or supplementation can keep homocysteine levels normal and significantly lower your risk of heart disease and other health problems such as reduced brain function. Folic acid is contained in many leafy vegetables, fruits, legumes, eggs and liver. Vitamin B12 can be obtained by eating fish, meat and eggs. Vitamins B1 and B2 are also important for the heart and are contained in meats, eggs, legumes, seeds and vegetables.

### Eggs, Cholesterol Consumption and Heart Disease

Most people love the taste of eggs, whether fried, scrambled, poached, hard-boiled or in a fancy soufflé. And as discussed in chapter 13, eggs are one of the best sources of quality protein and also contain a wide variety of other important nutrients. But, as everyone knows, egg yolks contain cholesterol. Do you avoid eating eggs because you fear they will somehow raise your blood cholesterol to dangerously high levels? The fact is, eating eggs won't necessarily raise your total cholesterol, because cholesterol in your blood is not there due to what you ate; instead most of it is made by your liver. There are other issues to consider as well. Let's examine some of facts about eggs, cholesterol and health.

First, let's answer this question: Will eating too much dietary cholesterol raise your blood cholesterol? The scientific evidence indicates the answer is "no," unless you're one of the few people who can't metabolize this fat. If that's the case, most likely your cholesterol is already too high — above 250 or 300.

In most healthy people, the body has compensation mechanisms to keep cholesterol in balance, even when you eat whole eggs every day. Your body absorbs a lot less cholesterol than you consume, especially if you eat fiber-rich foods. A study published in the August 1999 issue of the *Journal of Lipid Research* reported a cholesterol-absorption rate of 41 percent when subjects were fed only 26 mg. However, when the subjects were fed 188 mg of cholesterol, just 36 percent was absorbed. When fed 421 mg — the equivalent of two eggs — the subjects absorbed only 25 percent of the cholesterol, far below the maximum recommended daily allowance of 300 mg.

If this isn't enough to quell your egg phobia, consider these points about consumption of eggs and other foods high in cholesterol:

- Data from the Framingham Study, the largest ongoing medical study, revealed no relationship between cholesterol consumption and blood levels in 16,000 participants tracked over the course of six years.

- The fat in egg yolks is nearly a perfect balance, containing mostly monounsaturated fats, and about 36 percent saturated fat. Monounsaturated fat has been shown to raise HDL cholesterol levels. Studies published in the *New England Journal of Medicine* and the *Journal of Internal Medicine* indicate that eating whole eggs daily significantly raised the good HDL cholesterol.

- Egg yolks contain linoleic and linolenic acids. A 1994 study at the Boston University School of Medicine showed that these essential fatty acids are as important as all other vitamins and minerals, and are crucial in the regulation of cholesterol. The study also showed that without these fats in your diet, your risk for heart disease is increased.

- Egg yolks are high in lecithin, which assists the action of bile from the gall bladder in regulating cholesterol. Cholesterase, an important enzyme in egg yolks, may also help control cholesterol.

With all this scientific evidence, there seems to be little logical reason to avoid eating eggs. But if that's not enough for you, consider the clinical case of the "Egg Man." As reported in the *New England Journal of Medicine*, and on popular talk shows, an 88-year-old man with a documented history of eating 25 eggs per day was evaluated and found to be in excellent health, including normal weight and no signs, symptoms or history of heart disease, stroke or gall-bladder problems. His serum cholesterol over the years has ranged from 150 to 200, despite the fact that he eats about 5,000 mg of cholesterol per day! He is an example of the fact that increasing cholesterol intake, even by significant amounts, may not affect serum cholesterol levels.

Many other professionals question the anti-egg and cholesterol campaigns and the connection of egg and cholesterol consumption to heart disease. Now the traditional across-the-board recommendation that all people restrict egg intake is not backed by many prestigious experts in the field; M.F. Oliver, M.D., writing in *Circulation*, says that rather than telling everyone to cut down on cholesterol, we should identify those most at risk and improve their lifestyles. Thomas Moore, author of *Heart Failure* (Simon & Schuster, 1990), writes that the health advice given to millions of Americans over several decades has been tested in a large and elaborate clinical trial, and has produced no measurable benefits. Thomas Chalmers, of Mt. Sinai Medical School and the Harvard School of Public Health, says: "They have made an unconscionable exaggeration of all the data." And finally, Ed Ahrens, Jr., professor at Rockefeller University, says, "I think the public is being hosed by the NIH [National Institutes of Health] and the American Heart Association."

Will egg phobia end soon? More people are realizing that eating eggs doesn't raise their cholesterol, and that consuming too many carbohydrates and hydrogenated fats can be much more of a risk factor for heart disease, because these lower the protective HDL and raise LDL. For people who still need more information to overcome their fears, visit the Egg Nutrition Center's website at http://www.enc-online.org.

**Hypertension and Sodium: Just Another Scare?**
The common notion that sodium causes high blood pressure is erroneous. In some people with existing high blood pressure, excessive sodium can magnify the

problem. But only about 30 to 40 percent of hypertensives are sodium-sensitive. For these individuals, even moderate amounts of sodium can increase their blood pressure further. Obviously, these people should regulate their sodium intake. But salt modification for those who have normal blood pressure is not necessary, as sodium will not raise blood pressure in normal individuals.

Sodium is a necessary nutrient, essential for good health. An average healthy man of 150 pounds has about 90 grams of sodium in his body. One-third of this is as part of healthy bones and most of the remaining two-thirds surrounds the cells throughout the rest of the body, where sodium is a major player in their regulation. Balanced with potassium, sodium acts as an "electrochemical pump" in accomplishing this remarkable feat.

Sodium also helps regulate the acid/alkaline balance, water balance, the heartbeat and other muscle contractions, sugar metabolism and even blood-pressure balance.

The problem of hypertension should not be taken lightly, as it is a serious health risk. But how is hypertension defined? Experts disagree on the definition of high blood pressure. In the United States, pressures of 140/90 mm Hg are often considered borderline hypertension and are sometimes medicated. But many doctors still consider those numbers at the high end of normal. In people over the age of about 60, these "normals" tend to be higher, up to 160/95, as blood pressure ordinarily rises with age. In Canada, physicians generally do not consider blood pressures up to 190/100 in the elderly a problem requiring medication. It's obvious that this situation is not black-and-white, and people must be treated individually.

Normally, everyone's blood pressure continually changes, and often is higher with more stress. At times, some people with normal pressures show more significant increases when at the doctor's office. This "white-coat hypertension," as it's been termed, is usually benign.

One factor does have general acceptance: Certain individuals, due to some problem in their kidneys and/or adrenals, are unable to process sodium normally. This results in increased blood pressure.

Despite the fact that the American Heart Association and the Surgeon General recommend sodium restriction to prevent hypertension, other equally valid scientific opinions disagree. The American Council on Science and Health states in its literature that "stronger evidence should be available before persons are advised to alter their diets, and further caution that the possibility of harmful effects [of sodium restriction] cannot be totally discounted."

### Other Factors Associated with Hypertension

Treatment of hypertension should include an attempt to find its cause. Two common reasons for high blood pressure include kidney problems and narrowed or "clogged" arteries. Other causes may be nutritional, especially carbohydrate intolerance, which is present in almost all patients with hypertension. When certain nutrients are low, such as calcium and vitamins A and C, the blood pressure may elevate. In other cases, emotional factors can play a primary role. A lack of exercise has also been linked to hypertension.

In the United States, more than $3 billion is spent annually for blood-pressure medication. Ideally, correcting hypertension without medication is the healthiest approach. But when drugs are required, the proper medication and dose, along with careful observation for side effects, is vital. Although high blood pressure is dangerous, lowering it too much is not without potential problems. The findings of Dr. Michael Alderman and co-workers of the Albert Einstein College of Medicine show that too much lowering of blood pressure may reduce blood flow to the heart, which can put the heart at risk. The safest approach is a 10 percent reduction in blood pressure in a person with hypertension.

Many people do not realize they can often control their own hypertension. Here are some examples:

- Exercise is a very important factor in controlling high blood pressure. Studies show non-exercising persons are 1.5 times more likely to develop hypertension than fit individuals. Even in children, higher blood pressures are seen in those most inactive. Not only does increased activity in children result in lower blood pressures, but those who are active in sports have a lower incidence of hypertension later in life.

- Hypertension has an association with dietary fats. Unfortunately, the common belief is that a low-fat diet lowers blood pressure. This is untrue. Actually, studies have shown just the opposite. Unsaturated vegetable oils can lower blood pressure in many individuals. In one study in the *American Journal of Cardiology* (1988), low levels of series 2 eicosanoids derived from B fats were related to the inability of the kidneys to eliminate salt, thus causing higher blood pressures.

- For those who are overweight, reducing weight can result in a drop in blood pressure. The prevalence of hypertension is 50 percent higher in overweight individuals. When weight is reduced, blood pressure also goes down. It's also known that children and adolescents who are overweight are much more likely to have high blood pressure as adults.

Obviously, there's more to assessing your risk of heart disease than just worrying about your cholesterol levels. Smoking, high blood pressure and obesity can increase risk significantly. But other factors such as carbohydrate intolerance, inflammation, nutritional imbalances and stress can put you at cardiovascular risk, too. When assessing cardiovascular risk, it is important to consider all these factors, as well as some not mentioned. It's also important to realize that the heart can repair itself — so even for those who have a history of heart problems, you can help the body's repair process by optimizing your health and fitness.

# 34 Beating the Cancer Odds

As a society we tend to be reactionary rather than proactive. We wait for the government's latest list of carcinogens to avoid, and go for annual checkups to see if we have a disease such as cancer. Just the word "cancer" strikes fear in most people. However, coming to terms with "the C-word" and how to prevent it before it manifests as a growth, tumor or other abnormality can help reduce the fear associated with this deadly disease.

The primary thrust in mainstream medicine is to detect cancer in its earliest stages, and then try to fight the disease through radical medical intervention such as chemotherapy, radiation, surgery, or some combination of these. This has improved survival statistics of those diagnosed with cancer in recent years, but has done nothing to reduce actual rates at which people develop the disease.

This is unfortunate because most cancers may be preventable. Rather than have your doctor detect cancer early, wouldn't it be better to have your doctor not detect cancer at all? Ideally you want to avoid developing cancer altogether. A logical plan for avoiding cancer is to make certain lifestyle adjustments, avoid dangerous chemicals, and eat as if you *already* have cancer or other diseases.

Some scientists say cancer is an environmental problem. We know there are three main causes of cancer from our environment. The first is free radicals, or oxygen free radicals, discussed in the following chapter. The second is nitrogen-containing chemicals including those created by barbecuing meat; actually, many foods produce these nitrogen compounds during cooking, and preventing overheating such as by turning your steak every minute can prevent much of this problem. The third environmental cause of cancer is inflammation, which we have discussed several times throughout this book. To better understand how simple it may be to prevent cancer, it's helpful to know how cancer evolves, from onset to metastases.

## How Cancer Evolves

In most cases, regardless of what triggers cancer, there are three phases that follow. In cancer's initiation phase, a normal cell is changed to an altered cell through a process called mutation. Early in this first step, for example, free radicals can outweigh antioxidants, triggering DNA alterations. It is in this initiation phase that a person may have the most control over the process through diet and nutrition.

The next step is the proliferation phase, in which the cancer cells rapidly multiply, partly as a result of increased blood vessels that support such rapid cell growth. At this point, the affected area is referred to as a tumor. Continuing to use free radicals as an example, these are also necessary for tumor growth to proceed; antioxidants can impair tumor growth at this stage. The influence of food in promoting tumor growth also begins in this phase. One common example is carbohydrate intolerance, which promotes tumor growth through the action of excess insulin. Excess estrogens may also promote tumor growth in the proliferation stage, as can overproduction of series 2 eicosanoids from A and B fats.

These first two stages of cancer evolution are also termed pre-cancerous or pre-malignant. They may be accompanied by signs or symptoms, and sometimes discovered through medical tests. But more often they go unnoticed. These two phases can last decades — typically up to 30 years or more. So you have plenty of time to eat right and avoid chemical stresses if you start early. These phases are your best chance to avoid cancer through diet, nutrition and lifestyle improvements.

The third step is the invasion phase. Here, tumor growth becomes more widespread, is more commonly accompanied by signs and symptoms, and is relatively easy to diagnose. In this phase the cancer can metastasize. While this is the most common time period in which people turn to nutrition for help, it is also the phase in which this approach is least effective. Not that diet and nutrition can't help a person in this phase of cancer. But relative to how much benefit a person can obtain with diet and nutrition in phases one and two, when the cancer can be avoided, it's the phase in which these measures have the least therapeutic value.

### How Foods Can Prevent Cancer

We want to know which vitamin pill prevents cancer, when in fact there is none. Pharmaceutical companies are even now looking for this magic pill — a silver bullet to stop cancer in the early stages. If they find it, it will be something that already exists in foods we should be eating regularly as part of a healthy diet.

Rather than any one nutrient that can be obtained from a pill, it's the combination of nutrients from a variety of healthy foods that is by far the best protection to keep cancer and other diseases from starting in the first place. While billions of dollars are being spent on research each year to find "the cure for cancer," nature already provides it.

About 25 percent of those who eat the fewest fruits and vegetables have approximately double the cancer rate compared to those with the highest intake of these cancer-fighting foods. More frightening is that 80 percent of American children and adolescents, and almost 70 percent of adults, do not eat five portions a day of these foods. The result is a significantly reduced intake of key nutrients that help prevent cancer. It's estimated that at least half the population obtains too little of these important nutrients.

Low levels of key nutrients such as vitamin B12 and folic acid, vitamin B6 and niacin, vitamins C and E, and zinc can actually damage cellular DNA in the same manner as radiation and carcinogenic chemicals in our food and environment. Among the benefits of these nutrients is cancer prevention.

But don't look for the answer in the popular high-dose synthetic vitamins — they won't work like real food. In some cases, they can actually contribute to cancer promotion. As mentioned in our discussion of dietary supplements in chapter 18, common vitamin C products are one such example, since they can cause the same type of DNA damage that leads to the development of cancer.

### Preventative Chemo

Many of the substances that control inflammation also are chemopreventive, or in other words, they contain chemicals that can prevent cancer. Inflammation may be the first step to cancer formation, and excess inflammatory chemicals promote tumor growth. In addition, inflammation-causing enzymes are also responsible for cancer activation.

The foods that control activity of these enzymes, and development of many cancers, include raw garlic, turmeric, ginger, sesame seed and citrus peel, along with EPA fish oil. Others include green and black tea, and red wine. If you don't consume these foods, or your health indicates a higher intake is necessary, real-food dietary supplements are a must.

It's been discovered that, coincidentally, many anti-inflammatory drugs such as aspirin and other NSAIDs are chemopreventive. While certain drugs may reduce the risk of cancer, many natural foods provide the same protection, influencing the same enzyme systems without side effects.

Remember that diet and nutrition are not the only key factors in preventing cancer. Others include controlling certain lifestyle stresses, such as smoking, poor aerobic function, high body fat, and excess hormones such as insulin and estrogens.

### Functional Screening Helps Fight Disease

Routine testing for disease is a hallmark of modern medicine, but falls short of true prevention. By the time you test positive for a disease such as cancer, you already have it. Unfortunately, some screening tests may pose additional serious health risks.

Certainly, there are some instances when finding a disease in its early stages results in prompt and successful resolution of a potentially life-threatening problem. But there are too many other times when the same type of evaluation results in more problems, including an increased risk of death. A suspicious growth in the lungs, for example, could ultimately lead to surgery, which may pose more risk of death than the growth itself, especially if it's benign, which is the case in most of these situations.

A hot item of discussion is colonoscopy — a procedure for detecting colon cancer recommended by many health professionals, the media and some celebrities. Colonoscopy, like most other tests, is a valuable evaluation when matched with an individual's need. However, the risks that accompany colonoscopy are significant. Perforation of the colon occurs in up to 30 of every 10,000 patients during this procedure, with death occurring in 1 in 10,000. But the death rate of colon cancer itself is only about 1.8 per 10,000.

Herein lies one of the stories left untold by the popular media. With these evaluations come real risk of injury and death. The harm could also come in the form of follow-up care, including unnecessary surgery or drugs, significant psychological stress, or the recommendation for yet more tests. Rather than screening the entire population, those at high risk should be the ones screened.

An option for everyone is to use low-risk, non-invasive screening practices such as blood, urine and saliva tests to reveal risk factors or functional problems. By revealing problems that can be corrected before they become a full-blown disease, these tests are much more effective screening procedures than other tests that are suited only for ruling out already-existing diseases. And there are virtually no health risks associated with these tests themselves.

Besides the type of tests already mentioned, examples include a CBC blood test to assess both red and white blood cells, and blood-chemistry profiles that measure substances such as blood sugar (glucose); proteins (globulin and albumin); fats (cholesterol and triglycerides); minerals (sodium, potassium, calcium, iron); liver enzymes, and others. In addition, a simple blood test for C-reactive protein measures chronic inflammation, a precursor to more serious problems including cancer and heart disease. Salivary hormone tests and certain urine tests can more accurately reveal functional adrenal problems than blood tests.

**A Cancer-Fighting Plan for Eating**

While it's now accepted that diet and nutrition can play a significant role in reducing the onset and progression of the majority of cancers, unfortunately this concept has only recently been accepted by mainstream health care. Traditional cancer therapies, therefore, do not effectively or fully utilize diet and nutrition.

A dietary plan that provides a balance of protein, carbohydrate and fat, as well as vitamins, minerals and phytonutrients from vegetables, fruits and other health-promoting foods, can dramatically reduce the risk of cancer. It is important to obtain these nutrients from real foods or from supplements made from real foods, as it is the combined benefits of these items, rather than any single vitamin or mineral, that reduces the risk.

So where do you begin with prevention? Most of the lifestyle, dietary and nutritional principles discussed throughout this book are those that will help you avoid cancer. After all, that's what you want to do — postpone onset of this deadly disease to after you've died some other way, preferably in your sleep after a long and healthy life. Here is a review to serve as a starting point in your quest to postpone cancer.

- Consume antioxidant foods and supplements. Most people don't eat enough vegetables, fruits and other antioxidant-rich foods. You should eat five or more servings daily. Other antioxidant-rich foods include nuts and seeds such as almonds and sesame seeds, soy, extra-virgin olive oil and fresh meats.

- Consume anti-inflammatory foods and supplements. Most people don't get enough omega-3 fats, such as those contained in ocean fish, and consume too much omega-6 fat, contained in most vegetable oils. Since many people are omega-3 deficient, supplements such as EPA fish oil or flaxseed oil may be necessary.

- Eat a rainbow of vegetables and fruits. This variety will ensure the presence of adequate micro- and phytonutrients to help control inflammation and provide antioxidants, fiber and other anti-cancer substances. Be sure to include cruciferous vegetables such as broccoli, cabbage and Brussels sprouts. Also choose vegetables and fruits with bright colors such as carrots, squash and tomatoes, and leafy greens for the variety of folic-acid compounds that are present in nature but not in synthetic-vitamin supplements. Berries are good sources of cancer-fighting natural substances too.

- Avoid environmental chemicals at home and work. This includes chemicals from household cleaners, cosmetics and toiletries, paints, and other chemicals stored within your home. They all leak toxic substances that get into your body. This is especially true if your garage is attached to your house since your car continuously gives off large amounts of chemicals from gas, oil and other agents. Many types of house plants help filter the air, as does sufficient cross-ventilation from at least two partially open windows.

- Control physical, chemical and mental/emotional stress. Reducing all forms of stress reduces the production of oxygen free radicals, which damage DNA, the first step in the formation of cancer.

## Vegetables and Fruits Help Prevent Cancer

Years of research about disease prevention and treatment have shown that vegetables and fruits are much more effective than traditional dietary supplements in preventing disease. Scientists now can say that phytochemicals in plants explain why people who consume large amounts of vegetables and fruits, in general, have less chronic disease. Here are some examples:

- Chinese research, reported in the *Journal of the National Cancer Institute,* shows that allium vegetables — onions, garlic, chives, shallots and scallions — may be an important factor in reducing the risk of intestinal cancers.

- Celery, cucumber, endive, parsley and radish contain powerful phytochemicals with cancer-preventive properties.

- Those who consume more raw and fresh vegetables, including leafy greens, carrots, broccoli, cabbage, lettuce, tomatoes and fresh fruits, have lower cancer rates.

- Foods high in natural phytoestrogens, such as soy, peanuts and yams, are associated with a lower risk of hormone-related cancers.

- Those with diets low in vegetables have higher cancer rates.

**The Skinny on Skin Cancer**

Do you avoid the sun or use chemical sunscreens because you fear skin cancer? The fact is, avoiding the sun can leave you at risk for other types of cancer, and using sunscreen may actually contribute to cancer itself.

Researchers now report that lack of sun poses a much more serious threat than skin cancer by dramatically increasing risk factors for breast, colon and ovarian cancer. After extensive examination of cancer-mortality rates in 506 geographic regions in Europe and North America, a study published in the journal *Cancer* suggests that the likely trigger for these digestive- and reproductive-system cancers is low levels of ultraviolet B light, essential for the body to produce vitamin D. Naturally produced vitamin D protects against these types of cancer, while vitamin D from supplements has not been shown to be effective. The study also linked 25 percent of the breast cancer in Europe to insufficient sunlight exposure, and found rates of cancers of the reproductive and digestive systems twice as high in the New England states as the sunny southwest, despite similar dietary habits. Other cancers related to lack of natural vitamin D due to decreased sunlight exposure include those of the bladder, uterus, esophagus, rectum and stomach.

Furthermore, researchers projected that Americans would experience 85,000 additional cases and 30,000 additional deaths in 2002 from digestive- and reproductive-system cancers that otherwise would be prevented if all residents received the same amount of sun as those who live in the southern tier of states. While this additional sunlight exposure would lead to 3,000 additional skin-cancer deaths, it would result in 27,000 fewer cancer deaths overall.

These cases of skin cancer may be primarily among people who are not healthy enough to tolerate normal sun exposure. Your body is meant to absorb sunlight. But it's important to follow certain common-sense and dietary habits in order to do so in a healthy manner.

First, avoid sunburn. This does not mean slathering on the sunscreen, which may actually cause skin cancer, but rather limit exposure to the sun while you gradually build up your natural tan. Tanning is the body's natural defense against sunburn and skin cancer.

Second, be mindful of your diet and how this affects your skin and its reactions to the sun. Certain antioxidants, phytonutrients and oils have a profound effect on how your body reacts to sunshine. Naturally occurring antioxidants from foods and supplements made from real food, including vitamins C and E, the carotenoids, selenium, and the phytonutrient lycopene, help protect both the skin and eyes from damaging effects of the sun. Folic acid is also important since significant losses of this vitamin occur during sun exposure. However, these same nutrients obtained from high-dose synthetic and isolated dietary supplements may not offer as much protection.

There are also several factors to consider about dietary fats and sunshine. The most prevalent fat in the typical American diet is vegetable oil, such as soybean, corn and safflower oils. Too much of these oils in the skin can cause excessive free-radical stress—a first step in cancer formation. However, other fats have protective properties. Citrus-peel oil contains limonene, a phytonutrient that has been shown to help prevent and treat skin cancer. In addition, omega-3 fats offer ultraviolet protection and can help control inflammation, which may be a trigger to skin cancer.

Many people use sunscreen to prevent cancer. Actually, sunscreen may promote cancer in two ways. First, using sunscreen when spending a lot of time in the sun gives people the false sense that it's OK to stay in the sun for longer periods of time. Since sunscreen won't block all the sun's rays, increased exposure increases your risk of sun damage. Second, there is a relationship between the chemicals used in sunscreen and cancer development.

Early in their development, sunscreens contained PABA (para-aminobenzoic acid) to absorb sunlight, but these sunscreens disappeared from the market when it was learned that this substance causes DNA damage. Subsequent products were found to promote free radicals, which also contribute to cancer. The latest sunscreens contain elements such as titanium dioxide or zinc oxide to scatter or reflect sunlight, but unfortunately these chemicals also form free radicals on the skin; titanium dioxide has been linked to DNA damage as well.

The next generation of sun-protection products may simply be natural compounds such as antioxidants, carotenoids, flavonoids, phytonutrients and essential fatty acids. These, coupled with a good tan and common sense when it comes to sun exposure, will do the most to prevent skin cancer.

The best treatment for cancer is preventing it altogether. By eating foods that have been shown to fight cancer, following an eating plan to reduce the risk of disease and making certain lifestyle adjustments, you could ward off the development of cancer in your lifetime.

# 35 Antioxidants, Disease Prevention and Aging

In 1775, a biochemist named Joseph Priestly wrote in *Discovery of Oxygen* about the importance of oxygen, and its dangers. Today, we are aware of oxygen's benefits, but many people don't realize its potential harm: the conversion of the stable $O_2$ molecule to its very unstable and destructive cousin, the superoxide or free radical. When this occurs inside the body, it can lead to serious health problems. Scientists now associate oxygen free radicals with every major chronic disease, including heart disease and cancer. Free radicals also play a major role in the aging process. Aging is the result of continuous reactions of the body's cells with free radicals. It is important to become aware of these potentially harmful substances, what increases their production and how to control them, in order to reduce the devastating effects of disease and control the process of aging.

## Free-Radical Stress

Normally, free radicals protect against harmful bacteria, viruses, chemical pollutants and even toxic substances produced within the body. However, in this chemical-saturated world, it is possible to produce too many free radicals. When this occurs, free radicals can react with and damage any cell in the body. The most vulnerable part of the cell is the part containing unstable polyunsaturated fats, as these fats are easily destroyed by free radicals. This destruction, called lipid peroxidation, is the first step in the disease process. For example, before LDL cholesterol can be stored in the coronary arteries, damage from lipid peroxidation must first take place. Lipid peroxidation also is the first step in any inflammatory process. It produces toxins capable of traveling throughout the body, creating damage anywhere. These toxins are known to be carcinogenic and even have the potential to cause genetic mutations.

Deleterious free-radical reactions are also referred to as oxidative stress. The cellular changes resulting from free-radical damage are what we know as aging. Increases in oxidative stress, whether from too much free-radical production, too little antioxidant activity, or both, speeds the aging process, sometimes significantly.

## Antioxidants to the Rescue

One way the body regulates free radicals is through chemical conversion to less harmful substances. This is accomplished by natural chemicals known as antioxidants. The most common of these antioxidant free-radical "scavengers" include vitamins A, C and E, beta-carotene, selenium, the bioflavanoids, and phytonutrients such as phenols. In addition, biothiols such as those contained in whey help the body produce its most powerful antioxidant substance, glutathione. The following is a list of the most potent antioxidants in order of their effectiveness. As you can see, many of the most powerful are not the most popular versions.

| | |
|---|---|
| Sulforaphan | Lipoic acid |
| Cysteine | Alpha-tocotrienol |
| Gamma-tocopherol | Alpha-tocopherol |
| Vitamin C | Lycopene |
| Beta-tocopherol | Beta-carotene |
| Zeaxanthin | Delta-tocopherol |
| Lutein | Canthaxanthin |
| Astaxanthin | Quercetin |
| Co-Q10 | |

It's not necessary to remember the names of these antioxidants, but you do need to remember to eat as many antioxidant-rich foods as possible. These include vegetables and fruits, berries, sesame seeds, soy, oats, nut butters and extra-virgin olive oil. Green tea and red wine are excellent sources of antioxidants. Meats, especially beef, contain significant amounts of certain antioxidants, as do products that contain whey. Of course there are now hundreds of antioxidant products available in pill, liquid and powder form. If needed, be sure to take only supplements made from whole foods containing natural phytochemicals. Early signs and symptoms of the need for more antioxidants may include lingering cold or flu, sensitivity to chlorine or other chemicals, and inflammation.

### Case History

*Alice was in her mid-30s, and had a variety of very vague problems. One of her previous doctors told me he thought she was a hypochondriac. She had joint pain, but only on some days, was sensitive to perfumes, soaps and other substances containing certain chemicals, and when she got a cold (a half-dozen a year), it would last two to three weeks. In addition, she had skin rashes that the dermatologist could not identify, had burning eye pain several times each week, and looked about 50 years old. Her unusual history, including the disillusionment of her past doctor, and my evaluations, led me to recommend some antioxidants. My dietary advice*

*included several servings of fresh vegetables and a couple of low-glycemic*
*fresh fruits each day. Within about 10 days, Alice was noticeably*
*improved. Within a month, most of her problems were, by her words, 80*
*percent better. A year later, she reported only one cold, lasting three to*
*four days. And, her friends were telling her she looked much younger; she*
*certainly felt it.*

**Exercise and Free-Radical Activity**
Different levels of exercise intensity can produce varying amounts of free radicals. Easy aerobic exercise, especially at the heart rate determined by the 180 Formula, produces little or insignificant amounts of free radicals, and this smaller amount is most likely well controlled through the body's natural defense system, especially if enough antioxidants are present.

Moreover, a well-developed aerobic system has its own antioxidant effect. Fat-burning and free-radical breakdown occur in the mitochondria contained within aerobic muscle fibers. Therefore, people in better aerobic shape are more capable of controlling free radicals compared to those who are out of shape. Studies indicate that those with a higher percentage of aerobic muscle fibers have more antioxidant production and therefore more antioxidant capabilities.

However, exercising at higher intensities or lifting weights can have the opposite effect. Such intense activity may produce more oxidative stress — some studies show a 120 percent increase over resting levels. This is the result of physical damage to muscles, lactic-acid production and higher oxygen uptake, which may increase tenfold during the activity. Higher injury rates are also associated with increased free-radical production. In addition, production of more anaerobic muscle fiber means less aerobic mitochondria for free-radical elimination.

**Reduce Exposure to Chemicals**
In addition to eating foods that contain antioxidants, and perhaps taking them in supplement form, you can reduce free-radical production by simply avoiding exposure to certain substances. Taking in chemical pollutants, via your lungs, skin or through food, increases free-radical production by the body. Keep your home and work environment as free from pollutants as possible. Here are some tips for cleaning up your environment:

- New building materials, even new carpet and furniture, may pollute the indoor air you breathe. If you've just done some remodeling, redecorating, or if you have tightly sealed your home to save on heating costs (thereby sealing potential pollutants inside), keep two windows open just a bit to let in fresh air and vent your environment.

- Clean out your attic, basement, closets or other area in which you may have stored potential pollutants, such as old cans of paint, aerosols and cleaners. There is constant leakage of vapors from these products. Store all needed chemical products in an outside garage or shed, and discard the items you don't need or want and those too old to use. If your garage is attached to the house, try to vent the garage, as your car leaks fumes from gasoline, oil and other chemicals.

- The best way to filter your indoor air is nature's way — plants! Besides being attractive, they are very effective, often more so than any mechanical filtering device. Through photosynthesis, plants absorb carbon dioxide along with other gases, including the chemicals given off from furniture, cleaners and insulation. The plant's leaves filter the air, and the roots break down toxic chemicals into less harmful ones with their natural bacteria and fungi. The best plants for the job include elephant ear and lacy tree philodendrons, golden pathos and the spider plant. Any green plant will work well. About 10 plants per 1,000 square feet of living space are adequate. That's one to three plants per room, depending on room and plant size.

- Dietary pollution is another factor to consider. Avoid the use of chemical products in foods, whenever possible, as well as fried and charred fats. These substances can generate excess free radicals. Certain natural foods in large amounts can also increase free-radical production. These include sassafras (used in root beer) and fresh black pepper. Be sure your diet is as complete and healthful as possible. This will provide you with all the antioxidant nutrients your body needs.

- Assess your need and desire for cosmetics, which contain fragrances and other potentially harmful chemicals. These include the many soaps in your house and office, deodorant, after-shave lotion, hair spray, mouth wash, etc.

Cleaning up your environment does not mean being obsessive, which can introduce even more damaging stress. Just do your best to make your environment as clean and safe as you possibly can. This, coupled with adequate intake of antioxidants and a regular aerobic exercise program, will help keep oxidative stress from causing disease and premature aging. In time we all will age. The trick is to do so gracefully and healthfully. This is the subject of the next chapter.

## Wearing Your Free Radicals

One of the most toxic substances you may be exposed to is the solvent used in dry cleaning. This chemical, perchloroethylene, or "perc," is classified as a hazardous air pollutant by the Environmental Protection Agency. It has been associated with cancer and kidney problems, and has a detrimental effect on the nervous system. Wearing freshly dry-cleaned clothing can be a danger since the residue of this chemical remains in the clothing after the dry-cleaning process. Whether it enters the body through skin pores or inhalation, it can produce a free-radical problem.

To avoid exposure to perc, avoid dry cleaning whenever possible. Many garments that say "dry clean only" can still be hand washed. Buy clothes that don't require dry cleaning. If you must dry clean, hang your garment outside for as long as possible — at least a day or more — to allow the perc to escape or until the "dry-cleaning smell" is gone. If you're lucky enough to have in your neighborhood a professional "wet cleaner," which uses only detergents and water, use this alternative — it's the future of the cleaning industry. Wet cleaners are common in Europe but not yet in the United States.

If you swim in chlorinated pools, you should know the chlorine stays in your swim suit long after you've left the pool. Chlorine will chemically deteriorate your swim suit much sooner than normal wear and tear, or even before you get tired of it. One way to solve both problems is to use a product called SuitSaver™. It's an antioxidant for your clothes, removing the residual chlorine trapped by your bathing suit. You keep the chlorine that evaporates from your bathing suit out of your environment — out of the air and off your skin.

# 36 Keys to Successful Aging

Almost all mammals on earth have a lifespan six times their skeletal maturity. If we apply this animal model to humans, who reach skeletal maturity at about age 20, we should expect to live, on average, to age 120.

In our society, the average human animal barely reaches four times his or her skeletal maturity. But with modern technology, natural hygiene, and the awareness of chemicals that speed the aging process, there will soon be hundreds of thousands of people in the United States over the age of 100. Will you be one of them? And if so, will you welcome it, considering what your quality of life might be? While there is a genetic aspect to how long you will live, there also are many lifestyle factors that may be even more important. How well you care for yourself from the earliest age has a significant impact on both the length and quality of your life.

As life expectancy rapidly increases in modern cultures, we'll soon have many centenarians. Unfortunately, most people don't think they'll live that long, and many actually hope they won't. Others, however, welcome the challenge and excitement of seeing a fifth-generation descendant graduate from some futuristic high school, perhaps home-schooled by a certain wise old great-great-great-grandparent.

But who wants to attend this celebration in a wheelchair, unaware of where you are, what the name of the descendant is, or who his or her parents are? If you do happen to live to 120 years young, you want to be fully functional. Throughout this book I have offered information and insight to help you improve and maintain fitness and health, to achieve optimal human performance and to avoid or postpone disease. It's no coincidence that all of these concepts also apply to successful and healthy aging.

The term "successful aging" is not a catchy phrase or new program. It's a very real concept with practical applications for people of all ages. Scientists note three common paths for people as they age. "Successful aging" results in a higher quality of life. "Usual aging" would be considered "average." "Diseased aging" results in low quality of life and slow death. Average is unacceptable, and diseased is no way to live or to die. The better you age, the higher your quality of life, the more productive you are throughout life, and the less likely you will die a slow death.

The younger you are, the more you can do to control how well you age. The older you are, the more you want to control aging. Regardless of your age now, your actions can have significant impact on the way you age. In my years of practice and research I have identified seven key factors that can have a direct and powerful impact on how successfully you age. As you read these keys to successful aging you might also notice that these are, not coincidentally, a review of many concepts that I have put forth in this book. If you weren't willing to embrace these ideas for your health when you read them the first time, perhaps viewing them in light of how they will affect you later in life will help you to decide to make healthy changes now. To refresh your memory, return to the appropriate chapters after finishing this one. While these seven keys to successful aging may be a review for many, they're also a wake-up call for others who set less-significant priorities for day-to-day living rather than living well today for a healthy life tomorrow.

**Brain Nutrients**
The brain relies on many nutrients for normal function and aging. Among the most important are vitamins B6, B12, and folic acid, and omega-3 fats. These nutrients can help prevent Alzheimer's disease and similar conditions that are becoming very prevalent in the United States, as discussed later in this chapter.

Vitamins B6 and B12, and folic acid also happen to be three very important nutrients for preventing heart disease, stroke and peripheral vascular disease. And for the same reason — they prevent the rise of homocysteine levels in the blood. This amino acid is toxic to the brain. If you do not eat enough foods high in these nutrients, including meat, eggs, leafy vegetables, and fruits, supplementation may be necessary. Furthermore, high doses are not needed, but sufficient hydrochloric acid is necessary to aid in absorption of these nutrients.

**Anti-Inflammatory Foods**
Inflammation is a first step in the progression of heart disease, cancer and many other conditions. It also may be one of the main reasons too many people age poorly. A variety of foods have significant anti-inflammatory effects, including omega-3 fats, garlic, ginger, sesame, citrus peel and turmeric. Unfortunately, people eat much too little of these protective foods and overeat foods that can promote inflammation, especially vegetable oils and dairy products such as cream, milk and butter.

Other factors, including stress, hydrogenated oils, excess sugar and carbohydrates, can also promote inflammation. Unless sufficient anti-inflammatory foods are consumed, supplementing with omega-3 oils and other natural anti-inflammatory foods is essential to successful aging.

## Antioxidant Foods

Free-radical stress is another significant cause of poor aging. The standard recommendation to eat a diet high in vegetables and fruits provides extensive health benefits due to naturally occurring antioxidants and other nutrients in these foods. This requires consuming five, six, seven or more servings of high-quality vegetables each day — something most people don't do. Without adequate antioxidants, aging cannot proceed successfully.

Antioxidants don't just include the traditional vitamin A and/or beta-carotene, vitamin C, and vitamin E, but many other associated phytonutrients and substances, such as biothiols in whey, that have antioxidant effects. Obtaining these from foods or food-source supplements is key since the traditional synthetic antioxidant supplements have not been shown to be as effective as the real thing. This is because these products are severely lacking in therapeutic components. For example, almost all antioxidant supplements contain vitamin E as alpha-tocopherol, but almost none include tocotrienols — a vital part of the whole vitamin E complex that is 50 times more potent an antioxidant.

## Blood-Sugar Control

Controlling blood sugar can improve aging in at least two ways. It provides necessary fuel for the brain, with poor blood-sugar control being associated with Alzheimer's disease and similar conditions. Poor blood-sugar control also triggers significant stress via the adrenal-gland mechanisms. This can affect any existing weakness or vulnerability in the body including problems with the heart, blood vessels, or pancreas, resulting in heart attack, stroke or diabetes.

Blood sugar is best controlled with a healthy diet that matches your particular needs. For many people, this means eating more often than the traditional two or three meals a day — typically five or six smaller meals or snacks each day is best. This can help you burn more body fat and lower cholesterol.

## Protein

The body requires significant amounts of protein to meet many daily needs. We tend to think of protein as something only athletes need. But muscle function is a primary health factor in people of all ages. With aging comes reduced muscle mass, partly due to less physical activity. Increased protein in the diet amplifies the effect of physical activity. Studies also show that healthy aging is associated with protein intakes much higher than the current recommendations.

Protein foods such as meat, fish, eggs, whey and soy may be the best choices, with almonds and other nuts providing lesser amounts.

### Physical and Mental Activity

About 40 percent of people over the age of 50 are totally inactive — and half of these inactive people actually believe they get enough physical activity to keep fit. Worse yet, too many caregivers, from relatives to professionals, avoid recommending activity for fear of falls and other injuries. But the fact is, even for the most frail elderly, the risks associated with inactivity are greater than those associated with being active.

For those who are not naturally physically active, the addition of some type of regular activity is necessary for successful aging. This can include walking, swimming, using a stationary apparatus, or other type of aerobic activity, even if only a few minutes each time. If there has been a significant loss of muscle mass, lifting very light weights can help restore muscle function, balance and strength. This often allows some to add even more activity.

> **How Old Are You?**
> We all know people who appear much older, or younger, than their actual chronological age. While we tend to measure age by years — this is called chronological age — a person's physiological condition is a better indicator of actual age. This can actually be measured with tests for breathing, blood sugar, muscle function and others. Having the body and mind of a 40-year-old person when you're chronologically 60 is a real possibility.

### Emotional and Social Health

Successful aging can include many factors, and I have not forgotten about the issues involving a person's mental and emotional health. The need to socialize, to feel good about life, and other factors are so important for successful aging. While volumes have been written about this subject, my contention is that when people take the necessary steps to better health, they feel better mentally and emotionally, and tend to socialize more, which leads to better overall mental health.

### Improving Your Odds

Don't forget that we're all individuals with specific needs. There are unlimited possibilities, most of which are not listed here, but many of which have been addressed throughout this book. For example, many people don't get enough sun, or enough sleep, both of which can have a significant impact on aging. There are hundreds of similar examples that, taken in a specific combination, make up your unique set of needs. However, the major factors discussed above serve as a common starting point for most people in their quest to age successfully. In addition, here are some other tips to help you improve your chances for successful aging.

- Avoid "new" breakthroughs in food technology. Remember all those items now banned or discontinued because of the problems they created? New items are continually brought to market with a splash — but often removed in a shroud of secrecy. This especially includes fake foods, hot new diets and other items you hear about almost daily. Keep your guard up.

- Be skeptical of new over-the-counter and prescription drugs. Especially avoid those that were prescription at one time, but are now available in grocery-store aisles. The same is true for medical procedures. Take advantage of modern medicine by educating yourself about relevant issues, get numerous opinions, and avoid health professionals who won't take the time to talk with you (not at you).

- Watch out for potentially harmful dietary supplements. Many of these are really drugs in disguise. Examples include synthetic and isolated vitamins and minerals in doses that are higher than natural, and herbs that have side effects or may interact with other supplements or drugs. Some dietary supplements can have significant long-term side effects. Focus on getting all your nutrients from your diet, but know when to augment it with real dietary supplements.

- Reduce or avoid your exposure to chemicals. These chemicals may be found in air, food, water, household cleaners, laundry products and toiletries (including cosmetics) and can increase the aging process. The environment is not perfectly clean, but by electing to avoid most chemicals you can significantly impact your present and future health. Buy certified-organic foods, grow your own, and know where foods originate.

- Go barefoot as often as possible. Sound odd? Mortality increases dramatically following hip fracture, and wearing modern athletic shoes

**Age Does Not Cause Disease**

The government, the medical establishment and others fear the aging population for one main reason — additional medical expenses incurred by older people will take money away from other programs.

These fears stem from two incorrect assumptions made by most people. The first is that age must be associated with disease, and the second is that old age must be associated with dependency. While each of these pairs of factors often occur together, these are conveniently translated into the idea that age causes disease, and age produces expensive dependency. With these assumptions comes the fear that caring for older people will cost more since they're dependent on the health-care system.

But the fact is, old age does not cause disease — the same problems that cause disease in younger people do so in the elderly. Blaming a lack of health on being old is the ultimate health-care cop-out. Another fact is that older people with healthy habits live healthfully for longer periods of time. Dependency, or lack of it, is more often up to the individual. Healthy, fit aging is an option for those who seek it.

and shoes with high heels can increase the risk of fracture in older people. In addition, the generalized reduction in balance and stability from the long-term use of modern shoes results in reduced activity — something that can also lower your overall health.

- Be wary of modern electronics. Don't be afraid to use computers, cell phones, microwaves and other devices that may negatively impact your health, but limit their use. Avoid chatting on your cell phone, and when you need to use it do so with an extended antenna, or better yet, an ear-piece to avoid excessive electromagnetic stress. Use the microwave for that special dinner when you forgot to thaw the steak. Keep as far from your computer screen as possible. The effects of these devices are still not well known — assumptions that they don't cause harm are just not acceptable.

- Put your brain to work. Use it or lose it — learn to speak Japanese, take a course in astronomy or change careers regularly to keep your brain in tip-top shape. New hobbies such as painting, reading Einstein or any type of learning will force your brain to function better — even if you don't completely understand what you're reading. So as with your body, don't let your brain get out of shape. This also includes positive interactions with people you like, and avoiding those you don't — choose your friends wisely.

## Losing Your Mind?

Of all the problems people face with aging, deterioration of the mind (dementia) may be the most feared, with the various types of Alzheimer's disease being the cause in more than half these cases, afflicting 30 percent of those over age 85.

This degeneration of the brain begins much earlier in life — long before symptoms first appear. The key to successful treatment is to prevent the damage before it causes symptoms, since much of the damage may not be reversible. A number of dietary and nutritional factors can significantly aid in prevention, delaying onset and even treating this condition. Foremost among these are:

- Reducing chronic inflammation with omega-3 fats.

- Consuming appropriate natural B vitamins, including B12 and B6, as well as folic acid.

- Controlling free radicals through the use of antioxidants.

Getting these therapeutic nutrients begins with proper eating and supplementation, and also can be evaluated through various tests as discussed in their appropriate chapters.

### Indicators of Alzheimer's Are Many and Subtle

The earliest functional indicators of Alzheimer's are very subtle, and may include depression or emotional instability, lost sense of smell, general memory loss, long periods of low estrogen, decreased HDL cholesterol, increased adrenal stress hormones, and increased free radicals. Most of these problems can be remedied conservatively with diet, nutrition, stress reduction and exercise.

The earliest symptoms of Alzheimer's disease are much easier to observe, albeit more difficult to treat. The most common memory problem is lack of recall. Difficulty with numbers, such as balancing a checkbook, is also a common problem. Repeating statements and getting lost in a local area are less common but indicative of a more progressive problem, as is forgetting names of relatives or reductions in judgment.

**Will You Have an 'Optimal Death'?**
A Chinese proverb says we should all approach death with dignity. While living a long and healthy life past age 100, your physical and mental activity should be relatively high right up to the time of death — an event that should also be optimal. Perhaps on that day, you wake with the sunrise to a freshly made cup of Kona coffee. You settle in for a vegetable omelet and after reading e-mail from your children, grandchildren, great-grandchildren and their younger ones, you correspond to all. You spend some time writing in your diary, then head out for a long hike through the woods. After returning for a healthy lunch, you nap for an hour or so. You dawdle in the garden that afternoon, and follow that up with some easy paddling in the canoe. You watch the sun set with your significant other during a fine dinner complemented by a glass or two of Bordeaux, then share a piece of healthy but delicious chocolate. You head to bed, make love and fall asleep by 10:30. Just past midnight, you die peacefully during a sound sleep.

At the beginning of this book I described living a healthy life in terms of a 1,000-mile journey or race. Throughout I have put forth the ideas that I think will help you to achieve a lifetime of health, fitness and human performance. We are now at the end of this book but this is not the finish line. It's only the starting line. Throughout my life's journey, I plan on continuing my quest to "spread the word" about diet, nutrition, exercise, disease prevention and healthy living past age 100. Once again, I hope to see you at the finish line.

# References

Abernathy P et al. (1990). Acute and chronic responses of skeletal muscle to endurance and sprint exercise. Sports Med. 10(6):365-389.

Adachi H et al. (2000). Effects of Tocotrienols on Life Span and Protein Carbonylation in *Caenorhabditis elegans*. J Gerontol. 55A (6):B280-B285.

Adams P et al. (1996). Arachidonic acid to eicosapentaenoic acid ratio in blood correlates positively with clinical symptoms of depression. Lipids. 31:S157-S161.

Adler AJ et al. (1997). Effect of garlic and fish oil supplementation on serum lipid and lipoprotein concentrations in hypercholesterolemic men. Am J Clin Nutr. 65:445-450.

Ahrén B et al. (2001). The cephalic insulin response to meal ingestion in humans is dependent on both cholinergic and noncholinergic mechanisms and is important for postprandial glycemia. Diabetes. 50:1030-1038.

Aitken JC et al. (1989). The effects of dietary manipulation upon the respiratory exchange ratio as a predictor of maximum oxygen uptake during fixed term maximal incremental exercise in man. Eur J Appl Physiol. 58:722-727.

Aitken JC et al. (1988). The respiratory VCO2/VO2 exchange ratio during maximum exercise and its use as a predictor of maximum oxygen uptake. Eur J Appl Physiol. 57:714-719.

Almekinders L et al. (1993). Effects of repetitive motion on human fibroblasts. Med Sci Sports Exerc. 25(5):603-607.

Ames BN. (1998). Micronutrients prevent cancer and delay aging. Toxicology Letters. 102-103:5-18.

Arena B et al. (1995). Reproductive hormones and menstrual changes with exercise in female athletes. Sports Med. 19(4): 278-287.

Ascherio A et al. (1999). Relationship of consumption of vitamin E, vitamin C, and carotenoids to risk for stroke among men in the US. Ann Intern Med. 130:963-970.

Awad AB et al. (2000). Phytosterols as anticancer dietary components: evidence and mechanism of action. J Nutr. 130:2127-2130.

Barbeau WE. (1997). Interactions between dietary proteins and the human system: implications for oral tolerance and food-related diseases. Adv Exp Med Biol. 415:183-193.

Barrett J et al. (1995). The role of shoes in the prevention of ankle sprains. Sports Med. 20(4):277-280.

Bell J et al. (1996). Postexercise heart rates and pulse palpation as a means of determining exercising intensity in an aerobic dance class. Br J Sports Med. 30(1).48-52.

Bernton E et al. (1995). Adaptation to chronic stress in military trainees. Ann NY Acad Sci. 774:217-231.

Bird S et al. (1987). Pre-exercise food and heart rate during submaximal exercise. Br J Sports Med. 21(1):27-28.

Bjorntorp P. (1991). Importance of fat as a support nutrient for energy: metabolism of athletes. J Sports Sci. 9:71-76.

Black T et al. (2000). Palm Tocotrienols Protect ApoE +/- Mice from Diet-Induced Atheroma Formation. J Nutr. 130:2420-2426.

Blot W. (1997). Vitamin and mineral supplementation and cancer risk: international chemoprevention trials. Proc Soc Exp Biol Med. 216:291-296.

Bok S et al. (1999). Plasma and Hepatic Cholesterol and Hepatic Activities of 3-Hydroxy-3-methyl-glutaryl-CoA Reductase and Acyl CoA: Cholesterol Transferase Are Lower in Rats Fed Citrus Peel Extract or a Mixture of Citrus Bioflavonoids. J Nutr. 129:1182-1185.

Boone T et al. (1985). Carotid palpation at two exercise intensities. Med Sci Sports Exerc. 17(6):705-709.

Bosch A et al. (1993). Influence of carbohydrate loading on fuel substrate turnover and oxidation during prolonged exercise. J Appl Physiol. 74:1921-1927.

Boulay M et al. (1997). Monitoring high-intensity endurance exercise with heart rate and thresholds. Med Sci Sports Exerc. 29(1):125-132.

Bounous G. (2000). Whey protein concentrate and glutathione modulation in cancer treatment. Anticancer Res. 20(6C):4785-4792.

Brand-Miller JC et al. (1999). Evolutionary aspects of diet and insulin resistance. In: Simopoulos AP. Evolutionary aspects of nutrition and health. Diet, exercise, genetics and chronic disease. World Rev Nutr Diet. 84:74-105.

Brand-Miller JC et al. (2000). Insulin sensitivity predicts glycemia after a protein load. Metabolism 49(1):1-5.

Brandt K. (1987). Nonsteroidal antiinflammatory drugs and articular cartilage. J Rheumatol. 14:132-133.

Brizuela G et al. (1997). The influence of basketball shoes with increased ankle support on shock attenuation and performance in running and jumping. J Sports Sci. 15(5):505-515.

Broadhurst C. (1997). Balanced intakes of natural triglycerides for optimum nutrition: an evolutionary and phytochemical perspective. Med Hypotheses. 49(3):247-261.

Brouwer IA et al. (1999). Dietary Folate from Vegetables and Citrus Fruit Decreases Plasma Homocysteine Concentrations in Humans in a Dietary Controlled Trial. J Nutr. 129:1135-1139.

Christensen L et al. (1996). Comparison of nutrient intake among depressed and non-depressed individuals. Int J Eat Disord. 20(1):105-109.

Claassen N et al. (1995). The effect of different n-6/n-3 essential fatty acid ratios on calcium balance and bone in rats. Prostaglandins Leukot Essent Fatty Acids. 53(1):13-19.

Clark J et al. (1989). Viscoelastic shoe insoles: their use in aerobic dancing. Arch Phys Med Rehabil. 70(1):37-40.

Colliander E et al. (1988). Skeletal muscle fiber type composition and performance during repeated bouts of maximal, concentric contractions. Eur J Appl Physiol. 58:81-86.

Coulston A et al. (1993). Plasma glucose, insulin and lipid responses to high-carbohydrate low-fat diets in normal humans. Metabolism. 32:52-56.

Davalos A et al. (2000). Body iron stores and early neurologic deterioration in acute cerebral infarction. Neurology. 54(8):1568-1574.

David M et al. (1992). Effect of non-steroidal anti-inflammatory drugs (NSAIDS) on glycosyltransferase activity from human osteoarthritic cartilage. Br J Rheumatol. 31 (Suppl 1):13-17.

Dawson-Hughes B et al. (2002). Calcium intake influences the association of protein intake with rates of bone loss in elderly men and women. Am J Clin Nutr. 75(4):773-779.

Dieppe P et al. (1993). A two-year placebo-controlled trial of non-steroidal anti-inflammatory therapy in osteoarthritis of the knee joint. Br J Rheumatol. 32:595-600.

Donnelly A et al. (1990). Effects of ibuprofen on exercise-induced muscle soreness and indices of muscle damage. Br J Sports Med. 24:191-195.

Dueck C et al. (1996). Treatment of athletic amenorrhea with a diet and training intervention program. Int J Sport Nutr. 6(1):24-40.

Duncan B et al. (1995). Association of the waist-to-hip ratio is different with wine than with beer or hard liquor consumption. Am J Epidemiol.142:1034-1038.

The effect of vitamin E and beta-carotene on the incidence of lung cancer and other cancers in male smokers. The Alpha-Tocopherol Beta-Carotene Cancer Prevention Study Group (1994). N Engl J Med. 330(15):1029-1035.

Fabry P et al. (1970). Meal frequency – a possible factor in human pathology. Am J Clin Nutr. 23:1059-1068.

Fisher N et al. (1997). Muscle function and gait in patients with knee osteoarthritis before and after muscle rehabilitation. Disability and Rehabil 19(2):47-55.

Fisman E et al. (2001). Impaired fasting glucose concentrations in nondiabetic patients with ischemic heart disease: a marker for a worse prognosis. Am Heart J. 141(3):485-490.

Fontbonne A et al. (2001). Changes in cognitive abilities over a 4-year period are unfavorably affected in elderly diabetic subjects. Diabetes Care. 24:366-370.

Fruehwald-Schultes B et al. (2000). Adaptation of cognitive function to hypoglycemia in healthy men. Diabetes Care. 23:1059-1066.

Fry A et al. (1997). Resistance exercise overtraining and overreaching. Sports Med. 23(2):106-129.

Gardner L et al. (1988). Prevention of lower extremity stress fractures: a controlled trial of a shock absorbent insole. Am J Public Health. 78(12):1563-1567.

Glew RH et al. (2001). Cardiovascular disease risk factors and diet of Fulani pastoralists of northern Nigeria. Am J Clin Nutr. 74:730-736.

Golay A et al. (1996). Weight-loss with low or high carbohydrate diet? Int J Obes Relat Metab Disord. 20(12):1067-1072.

Goldberg L et al. (1988). Assessment of exercise intensity formulas by use of ventilatory threshold. Chest. 94(1):95-98.

Grace T et al. (1988). Prophylactic knee braces and injury to the lower extremity. J Bone Joint Surg. 70(3):422-427.

Graves J et al. (1988). Physiological responses to walking with hand weights, wrist weights, and ankle weights. Med Sci Sports Exerc. 20(3):265-271.

Guerrero-Romero F et al. (2001). Impaired glucose tolerance is a more advanced stage of alteration in the glucose metabolism than impaired fasting glucose. J Diabetes Complications. 15(1):34-37.

Guthrie N et al. (1997). Inhibition of Proliferation of Estrogen Receptor-Negative MDA-MB-435 and -Positive MCF-7 Human Breast Cancer Cells by Palm Oil Tocotrienols and Tamoxifen, Alone and in Combination. J Nutr. 127:544S-548S.

Halliwell B. (1998). Can oxidative DNA damage be used as a biomarker of cancer risk in humans? Problems, resolutions and preliminary results from nutritional supplementation studies. Free Radic Res. 29(6):469-486.

Han D et al. (1997). Protection against glutamate-induced cytotoxicity in C6 glial cells by thiol antioxidants. Am J Physiol. 273:R1771-R1778.

He L et al. (1997). Isoprenoids Suppress the growth of Murine B16 Melanomas In Vitro and In Vivo. J Nutr. 127:668-674.

Hertel J. (1997). The role of nonsteroidal anti-inflammatory drugs in the treatment of acute soft tissue injuries. J Athl Train. 32(2):350-358.

Hodgetts V et al. (1991). Factors controlling fat mobilization from human subcutaneous adipose tissue during exercise. J Appl Physiol. 71:445-451.

Holt S et al. (1997). An insulin index of foods: the insulin demand generated by 1000-kJ portions of common foods. Am J Clin Nutr. 66:1264-1276.

Horowitz J et al. (1994). High efficiency of type I muscle fibers improves performance. Int J Sports Med.15(3):152-157.

Hu FB et al. (1999). Nut consumption and risk of coronary heart disease: a review of the epidemiologic evidence. Curr Atherosclero Rep. 1:204-209.

Huang H et al. (2000). The effects of vitamin C and vitamin E on oxidative DNA damage: results from a randomized controlled trial. Cancer Epidemiol Biomarkers Prev. 9(7):647-652.

Jakes RW et al. (2001). Patterns of physical activity and ultrasound attenuation by heel bone among Norfolk cohort of European Prospective Investigation of Cancer (EPIC Norfolk): population based study. BMJ.322:140-143.

Jenkins DJ. (1997). Carbohydrate tolerance and food frequency. Br J Nutr. 77:S71-S81.

Jeppesen J et al. (1997). Effects of low-fat, high-carbohydrate diets on risk factors for ischemic heart disease in postmenopausal women. Am J Clin Nutr. 65(4):1027-1033.

Jorgensen U. (1990). Body load in heel-strike running: the effect of a firm heel counter. Am J Sports Med. 18(2):177-181.

Khan MI. (1997). Fracture healing: role of NSAIDs. Am J Orthop. 26(6):413.

Kincherf R et al. (1996). Low plasma gluta-mine in combination with high glutamate levels indicate risk for loss of body cell mass in healthy individuals. J Mol Med. 74:393-400.

Kirwan J et al. (1988). Physiological response to successive days of intense training in competitive swimmers. Med Sci Sport Exer. 20:255-259.

Koh KK et al. (2002). Statin attenuates increase in C-reactive protein during estrogen replacement therapy in post-menopausal women. Circulation. 105(13):1531-1533.

Korol DL et al. (1998). Glucose, memory, and aging. Am J Clin Nutr. 67:764S-771S.

Kris-Etherton P et al. (2001). The effects of nuts on coronary heart disease risk. Nutr Rev. 59(4):103-111.

Kris-Etherton P et al. (1999). High-monoun-saturated fatty acid diets lower both plasma cholesterol and triacylglycerol concentrations. Am J Clin Nutr.70:1009-1015.

Krivickas LS. (1997). Anatomical factors associated with overuse sports injuries. Sports Med. 24(2):132-146.

Kuipers H. (1994). Exercise-induced muscle damage. Int J Sports Med. 15(3):132-135.

Laio D et al. (2001). Abnormal glucose tolerance and increased risk for cardiovascular disease in Japanese-Americans with normal fasting glucose. Diabetes Care. 24:39-44.

Lambert E et al. (1994). Enhanced endurance in trained cyclists during moderate intensity exercise following 2 weeks adaptation to a high fat diet. Eur J Appl Physiol. 69:287-293.

Lands LC et al. (1999). Effect of supplementation with a cysteine donor on muscular performance. J Appl Physiol. 87(4):1381-1385.

Lands LC et al. (2000). Total plasma antioxidant capacity in cystic fibrosis. Pediatr Pulmonol. 29(2):81-87.

Leanderson J et al. (1993). Ankle injuries in basketball players. Knee Surg Sports Traumatol Arthrosc. 1(3-4):200-202.

Lee SH et al. (2001). Vitamin C-Induced Decomposition of Lipid Hydroperoxides to Endogenous Genotoxins. Science. 292(5524):2083-2086.

Lehmann M et al. (1997). Training and overtraining: an overview and experimental results in endurance sports. J Sports Med Phys Fitness. 37:7-17.

Lemon PW (1996). Is increased dietary protein necessary or beneficial for individuals with a physically active lifestyle? Nutr Rev.54 (4 Pt 2):S169-S175.

Leo M et al. (1999). Alcohol, vitamin A, and ß-carotene: adverse interactions, including hepatotoxicity and carcinogenicity. Am J Clin Nutr. 69:1071-85.

Liu G et al. (1983). Effect of high-carbohydrate-low-fat diets on plasma glucose, insulin and lipid responses in hypertriglyceridemic humans. Metabolism. 32(8):750-753.

Mayer A. (1997). Historical changes in the mineral content of fruits and vegetables: A cause for concern? Br Food J. 99:207-211.

McGrath SA et al. (1994). The effects of altered frequency of eating on plasma lipids in free-living healthy males on normal self-selected diets. Eur J Clin Nutr. 48:402-407.

Meagher EA et al. (2001). Effects of Vitamin E on Lipid Peroxidation in Healthy Persons. JAMA. 285:1178-1182.

Meigs JB et al. (1998). Metabolic risk factors worsen continuously across the spectrum of nondiabetic glucose tolerance. Ann Intern Med. 128:524-533.

Micke P et al. (2001). Oral supplementation with whey proteins increases plasma glutathione levels of HIV-infected patients. Eur J Clin Invest. 31(2):171-178.

Minet JC et al. (2000). Assessment of vitamin B-12, folate, and vitamin B-6 status and relation to sulfur amino acid metabolism in neonates. Am J Clin Nutr. 72:751-7.

Mitrakou A et al. (1991). Hierarchy of glycemic thresholds for counterregulatory hormone secretion, symptoms, and cerebral dysfunction. Am J Physiol. 260(1Pt1):E67-E74.

Moller P et al. (1996). Oxidative stress associated with exercise, psychological stress and life-style factors. Chem Biol Interact. 102(1):17-36.

Muoio D et al. (1994). Effect of dietary fat on metabolic adjustments to maximal VO2 and endurance in runners. Med Sci Sports Exerc. 26(1):81-88.

Nestler J. (1994). Assessment of insulin resistance. Sci AM: Sci & Med. 1(Sept/Oct):58-67.

Newsholme E. (1994). Biochemical mechanisms to explain immunosuppression in well-trained and overtrained athletes. Int J Sports Med 3:S142-S147.

Nieman DC. (1997). Immune response to heavy exertion. J Appl Physiol. 82(5):1385-1394.

NutrAnalysis, Inc., P.O. Box 306, Lake Lure, NC 28746. (800) 377-7978.

Omenn GS et al. (1996). Effects of a combination of beta carotene and vitamin A on lung cancer and cardiovascular disease. N Engl J Med. 334:1150-5.

Ostlund RE et al. (1999). Cholesterol absorption efficiency declines at moderate dietary doses in normal human subjects. J. Lipid Res. 40:1453-1458.

Packer L et al. (2001). Molecular Aspects of alpha Tocotrienol Antioxidant Action and Cell Signaling. J Nutr. 131:369S-373S.

Pan D et al. (1995). Skeletal muscle membrane lipid composition is related to adiposity and insulin action. J Clin Invest. 96:2802-2808.

Pendergast DR et al. (2000). A perspective on fat intake in athletes. J Am Coll Nutr. 19(3):345-50.

Pendergast DR et al. (1996). The role of dietary fat on performance, metabolism, and health. Am J Sports Med. 24(6):S53-S58.

Petroni A et al. (1997). Inhibition of leuko-cyte leukotriene B4 production by an olive oil-derived phenol identified by mass-spec-trometry. Thromb Res. 87(3):315-322.

Qureshi A et al. (1996). Dietary alpha toco-pherol attenuates the impact of gamma tocotrienol on hepatic 3-hydroxy-3-methyl-glutaryl coenzyme A reductase activity in chickens. J Nutr. 126:389-394.

Qureshi A et al. (1991). Dietary tocotrienols reduce concentrations of plasma choles-terol, apolipoprotein B, thromboxane B2, and platelet factor 4 in pigs with inherited hyperlipidemias. Am J Clin Nutr. 53:1042S-1046S.

Qureshi A et al. (1991). Lowering of serum cholesterol in hypercholesterolemic humans by tocotrienols. Am J Clin Nutr. 53:1021S-1026S.

Qureshi A et al. (1995). Response of hyperc-holesterolemic subjects to administration of tocotrienols. Lipids. 30:1171-1177.

Rieck J et al (1999). Urinary loss of thiamine is increased by low doses of furosemide in healthy volunteers. J Lab Clin Med. 134:238-243.

Robbins S et al. (1997). Balance and vertical impact in sports: role of shoe sole materi-als. Arch Phys Med Rehabil. 78(5):463-467.

Robbins S et al. (1998). Factors associated with ankle injuries. Sports Med. 25(1):63-72.

Robbins S et al. (1997). Hazard of deceptive advertising of athletic footwear. Br J Sports Med. 31(4):299-303.

Robbins S et al. (1987). Running-related injury prevention through barefoot adapta-tions. Med Sci Sports Exerc. 19(2):148-156.

Safran M et al. (1989). Warm-up and muscular injury prevention. An update. Sports Med. 8(4):239-249.

Salonen J. (1992). High stored iron levels are associated with excess risk of myocardial infarction in eastern Finnish men. Circula-tion. 86:803-811.

Selhub J et al. (2000). B vitamins, homocys-teine, and neurocognitive function in the Elderly. Am J Clin Nutr. 71:614S-620S.

Sen C et al. (2000). Molecular Basis of Vitamin E Action. J Biol Chem. 275(17):13049-13055.

Sen C et al. (2000). Thiol homeostasis and supplements in physical exercise. Am J Clin Nutr. 72:653S-69S.

Siguel E (1995). Does linoleic acid contribute to coronary artery disease? Am J Clin Nutr. 61(2):397.

Simi B et al. (1991). Additive effects of train-ing and high-fat diet on energy metabo-lism during exercise. J Appl Physiol. 71(1):197-203.

Simoneau J et al. (1985). Human skeletal muscle fiber type alteration with high-intensity intermittent training. Eur J Appl Physiol. 54:250-253.

Skouby SO et al. (1990). Mechanism of action of oral contraceptives on carbohydrate metabolism at the cellular level. Am J Obstet Gynecol. 163:343-348.

Solomons NW. (1986). Competitive interaction of iron and zinc in the diet: consequences for human nutrition. J Nutr. 116(6):927-935.

Strachan M et al. (2001). Acute hypoglycemia impairs the functioning of the central but not pheripheral nervous system. Physiol Behav. 72(1-2):83-92.

Suter P et al. (2000). Diuretic and Vitamin B1: Are diuretics a risk factor for thiamin mal-nutrition? Nutr Rev. 58(10):319-323.

Tan D et al. (1991). Effect of a palm oil vitamin E concentrate on the serum and lipoprotein lipids in humans. Am J Clin Nutr. 53:1027S-1030S.

Tchernof A et al. (2002). Weight Loss Reduces C-Reactive Protein Levels in Obese Postmenopausal Women. Circulation. 105:564.

Theriault A et al. (1999). Tocotrienol: A Review of Its Therapeutic Potential. Clin Biochem. 32(5):309-319.

Titan SM et al. (2001). Frequency of eating and concentrations of serum cholesterol in the Norfolk population of the European prospective investigation into cancer: cross sectional study. BMJ. 323:1-5.

Tomaro J et al. (1993). The effects of foot orthotics on the EMG activity of selected leg muscles during gait. J Orthop Sports Phys Ther. 18(4):532-536.

Towler D et al. (1993). Mechanism of awareness of hypoglycemia. Perception of neurogenic (predominantly cholinergic) rather than neuroglycopenic symptoms. Diabetes. 42(12):1691-1693.

Urhausen A et al. (1997). Blood hormones as markers of training stress and overtraining. Sports Med. 20(4):251-276.

Vea H et al. (1992). Reproducibility of glycaemic thresholds for activation of counterregulatory hormones and hypoglycaemic symptoms in healthy subjects. Diabetologia. 35(10):98-961.

Vegt F et al. (2001). Relation of impaired fasting and postload glucose with incident type 2 diabetes in a Dutch population. JAMA. 285:2109-2113.

Venkatraman JT. (1998). Effects of the level of dietary fat intake and endurance exercise on plasma cytokines in runners. Med Sci Sports Exerc. 30(8):1198-1204.

Vinson JA et al. (1988). Comparative bioavailability to humans of ascorbic acid alone or in a citrus extract. Am J Clin Nutr. 48:601-604.

Wagner EH et al. (2001). Effect of improved glycemic control on health care costs and utilization. JAMA. 285:182-189.

Weyer C et al. (2001). Insulin resistance and insulin secretory dysfunction are independent predictors of worsening of glucose tolerance during each stage of type 2 diabetes development. Diabetes Care. 24:89-94.

Wilkinson TJ et al. (1997). The response to treatment of subclinical thiamine deficiency in the elderly. Am J Clin Nutr. 66(4):925-928.

Woo OF et al (2000). Shorter duration of oral N-acetylcysteine therapy for acute acetaminophen overdose. Ann Emerg Med. 35(4):363-368.

Worthington V. (2001). Nutritional Quality of Organic Versus Conventional Fruits, Vegetables, and Grains. J Alt Comp Med. 7(2):161-173.

Yu W et al. (1999). Induction of apoptosis in human breast cancer cells by tocopherols and tocotrienols. Nutr Cancer. 33(1):26-32.

Zeisel SH. (1999). Regulation of "nutraceuticals." Science. 285:1853-1855.

# Index

# Other Books and Booklets
## by Dr. Phil Maffetone

*Training for Endurance*

*Eating for Endurance*

*Complementary Sports Medicine*

In addition to these books, Dr. Maffetone has written
the *ABCs* series of informational booklets
on various health topics, including fat-burning,
weight loss, inflammation, hormonal stress
and executive endurance.

For information about these books, booklets,
or products mentioned in this book,
contact MAF BioNutritionals.

*The Maffetone Report* bimonthly newsletter
explores timely health-related topics.
Contact MAF BioNutritionals
for subscription information.

Toll-free (877) 264-2200

www.mafbionutritionals.com